W

Therapeutic Communication

FOR HEALTH CARE PROFESSIONALS

Fourth Edition

Therapeutic Communication

FOR HEALTH CARE PROFESSIONALS

Fourth Edition

Carol D. Tamparo

BS, PhD, CMA-AAMA
Former Dean of Business and Allied Health,
Lake Washington Institute of Technology,
Kirkland, Washington

Wilburta Q. Lindh

CMA-AAMA
Professor Emerita,
Highline College,
Des Moines, Washington

LIS - LIBRARY

Date	Fund
17/2/20	nm-LEI

Order No.

2985 482

University of Chester

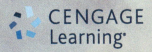

CENGAGE
Learning·

Australia • Brazil • Japan • Korea • Mexico • Singapore • Spain • United Kingdom • United States

JET LIBRARY

CENGAGE
Learning™

**Therapeutic Communication
for Health Care Professionals,
Fourth Edition**

Carol D. Tamparo and Wilburta Q. Lindh

SVP, GM Skills & Global Product
Management: Dawn Gerrain

Product Director: Matthew Seeley

Product Manager: Laura Stewart

Senior Director, Development:
Marah Bellegarde

Senior Product Development Manager:
Juliet Steiner

Content Developer: Kaitlin Schlicht

Product Assistant: Deb Handy

Vice President, Marketing Services:
Jennifer Ann Baker

Marketing Manager: Jessica Cipperly

Senior Production Director: Wendy
Troeger

Production Director: Andrew Crouth

Senior Content Project Manager:
Betty Dickson

Senior Art Director: Jack Pendleton

Cover image: ©nature photos/
ShutterStock.com

For product information and technology assistance, contact us at
**Cengage Learning Customer & Sales Support,
1-800-354-9706**

For permission to use material from this text or product,
submit all requests online at **www.cengage.com/permissions**.
Further permissions questions can be e-mailed to
permissionrequest@cengage.com

Library of Congress Control Number: 2016930484

ISBN: 978-1-305-57461-8

Cengage Learning
20 Channel Center Street
Boston, MA 02210
USA

Cengage Learning is a leading provider of customized learning
solutions with employees residing in nearly 40 different countries
and sales in more than 125 countries around the world. Find your local
representative at **www.cengage.com**.

Cengage Learning products are represented in Canada by Nelson
Education, Ltd.

To learn more about Cengage Learning, visit **www.cengage.com**
Purchase any of our products at your local college store or at our
preferred online store **www.cengagebrain.com**

Printed at CLDPC, USA, 10-19

Dedication

This book is dedicated to every instructor, professor, student, or health care professional who recognizes and practices the all-important component of comprehensive health care—therapeutic communication. It is also dedicated to supportive and helpful husbands—Tom Tamparo and DeVere Lindh—who added helpful suggestions, carried the laptops on vacations, and encouraged us just at the right time.

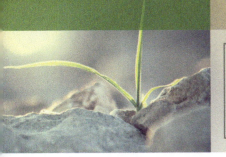

Contents

Chapter 2   Multicultural Therapeutic Communication 34

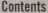

Chapter 5   The Therapeutic Response across the Life Span 108

Chapter 6 | The Therapeutic Response to Stressed, Anxious, and Fearful Clients 134

Chapter 7   The Therapeutic Response to Angry, Aggressive, Abused, or Abusive Clients 162

Chapter 10 — The Therapeutic Response to Clients with Life-Altering Illness 230

Chapter 11 — The Therapeutic Response to Clients Experiencing Loss, Grief, Dying, and Death 248

Appendix A   Theories of Human Growth and Development 268

Appendix B   Defense Mechanisms 288

Preface

Therapeutic Communication for Health Care Professionals, Fourth Edition is a critical and key component of health care for any client. Today's climate of health care is both technical and clinical. Because interaction with clients and patients can often be rushed, the client may be left feeling devalued and with many unanswered questions. This text addresses the critical need in health care today for successful therapeutic communication between health care staff and clients. Effective communication with clients can decrease stress, increase client compliance, and result in a positive experience for all involved. Members of all health care professions will benefit from the information in this text, including students of allied health programs and nursing programs.

Instructors at all levels of health care indicate that teaching "soft skills" like effective communication is one of the most difficult tasks they face in the classroom. Students in all areas of health care can be taught the clinical and technical skills with the right amount of instructional oversight and practice; teaching students how to respond therapeutically in all situations is more difficult to teach in a classroom setting.

Organization of the Text

The key to learning the soft skills is exposure to and the ability to think critically in the moment. This text introduces the reader to the purpose and reality of therapeutic communication in all types of settings. The first five chapters introduce students in how to communicate with multicultural clients, with clients embracing complementary or alternative therapies, and with clients of varying ages and circumstances, as well as health care peers and professionals. In the last six chapters, the reader will learn how to respond therapeutically to clients who are stressed, anxious, fearful, angry, aggressive, abused or abusive, and depressed or suicidal. Special attention is given to clients with substance use disorders or life-altering illnesses, and to clients experiencing loss, grief, dying, or death.

Features

The Fourth Edition of *Therapeutic Communication for Health Care Professionals* is designed to make the learning process as intuitive as possible. Here is a brief description of each feature and its intended use.

Chapter Objectives: Provided at the start of each chapter, *Chapter Objectives* may be used to guide learning and test key facts presented in the chapter. Use these objectives, together with review and *For Further Consideration* questions and *Exercises*, to test student understanding of the chapter's content.

Opening Case Study: An Opening Case Study puts chapter content into a real-world context, to provide a framework for learning.

Key Terms: All key terms appear in bold at the first occurrence for easy identification. The glossary provides definitions for all key terms.

Case Studies: The "real-world" case studies provided within each chapter serve as a springboard for discussion, provide food for thought, and can be a means to emphasize key points in the chapter. Through these case studies students will come to understand some of the stimulating challenges faced by health care professionals and gain insight into how these challenges are overcome.

Stop and Consider: The *Stop and Consider* feature occurs throughout the learning process and provides an opportunity for critical thinking discussions.

The Therapeutic Response: Each chapter focuses in on the therapeutic response to health care client situations, applying techniques discussed to specific situations and special client needs in health care.

Icons: Icons for *Self-Awareness, Culture, Legal,* and *Professionalism* information are interspersed throughout the chapters and highlight important topic reminders.

 Self-Awareness

 The Self-Awareness icon indicates how health care professionals become aware of their character, feelings, motives, and desires, and their reactions to circumstances around them.

 Cultural

 The Cultural icon refers to attitudes, customs, beliefs, races, etc. that distinguish one group from another group.

 Legal

 The Legal icon applies to any procedure, practice, circumstance, etc. that is based in law or has legal ramifications.

 Professionalism

 The Professionalism icon refers to how health care professionals demonstrate competence, accountability, participate in teamwork and shared responsibility, and how they place their "best foot forward" with clients.

Exercises: Exercises at the end of each chapter present interesting and interactive ways for learners to apply theory and skills presented in the chapter to specific environments and situations. These exercises are practical and help learners become confident in using knowledge and skills.

Review Questions: These questions test the learner's comprehension of the chapter with structured multiple-choice questions.

For Further Consideration: This feature provides opportunities for learners to think beyond the text. The understanding of chapter material, as well as personal insight and judgment, will be required to respond.

End-of-Chapter Case Studies: These case studies challenge learners to think through options for solving problems critically, using the skills and knowledge they just learned.

References and Resources: A list of references from the text and materials readers may wish to explore is provided at the end of each chapter.

New to This Edition

Always, in any new edition, each chapter has been reviewed and updated with current information pertinent to therapeutic communication for health care professionals. Updates to the Fourth Edition include the following:

- A new chapter, Therapeutic Communication in Complementary Medicine, provides examples of negative and positive components of both alternative and traditional therapies for medical care. Learners are guided to an understanding of "integrative medicine."

- An improved text design and four-color art program with more tables, graphics, updated cartoons, and photographs enhance the content by providing quick visual references.

- An increased number of case studies throughout the chapters provides students with more opportunities to see real-world applications of the content.

- Multicultural interaction is again emphasized in the text with new material and examples.

- Emphasis has been placed on therapeutic communication across the life span in varying situations, including growth and development, stress, depression, and suicide.

- Bullying is defined and its impacts are discussed.

- A discussion of appropriate therapeutic approaches for those left behind after a suicide is presented.

- Palliative and hospice care are discussed as they relate to life-altering and life-threatening illness. Recent legislation on assisted death is included in the discussion of death and dying.
- The new *Professionalism* icon (noted earlier) highlights key information on characteristics of professionalism, such as competence, accountability, teamwork, and responsibility.

Learning Package for the Student

MindTap

(Printed Access Code ISBN 978-1-305-57462-5)

(Instant Access Code ISBN 978-1-305-57464-9)

Therapeutic Communication for Health Care Professionals, 4e on MindTap is the first of its kind in an entirely new category: the Personal Learning Experience (PLE). This personalized program of digital products and services uses interactivity and customization to engage students, while offering instructors a wide range of choices in content, platforms, devices, and learning tools. MindTap is device agnostic, meaning that it will work with any platform or Learning Management System and will be accessible anytime, anywhere: on desktops, laptops, mobile phones, and other Internet-enabled devices.

This MindTap includes:

- An interactive eBook with highlighting, note-taking, and more
- Flashcards for practicing chapter terms
- Computer-graded activities and exercises
- Easy submission tools for instructor-graded exercises
- Video case studies and listening drills

Teaching Package for the Instructor

The following supplements are available to enhance the use of *Therapeutic Communication for Health Care Professionals* in the classroom:

Instructor Companion Website

(ISBN 978-1-305-57470-0)

Spend less time planning and more time teaching with Cengage Learning's Instructor Companion Website to accompany *Therapeutic Communication for Health Care Professionals, 4e.* As an instructor, you will have access to all of your resources online, anywhere and at any time. All instructor resources can be accessed by going to www.cengage.com/login to create a unique user log-in. The password-protected instructor resources include the following:

- An electronic *Instructor's Manual* that is packed with everything an instructor needs to be effective and efficient in the classroom. The Instructor's Manual includes complete answer keys to textbook questions, as well as expert answers to the case studies in the book. It also includes complete lesson plans with suggested media and other visual aids, a complete presentation of topic-by-topic outline, and a discussion of how to use the textbook features and supplements to your advantage in the classroom.
- Customizable PowerPoints® for each chapter.
- *Cengage Learning Testing Powered by Cognero*, which is a flexible, online system that allows you to author, edit, and manage test bank content from multiple Cengage Learning solutions; you can also create multiple test versions in an instant, and deliver tests from your learning management system (LMS), classroom, or elsewhere.

MindTap

(Printed Access Code ISBN 978-1-305-57462-5)

(Instant Access Code ISBN 978-1-305-57464-9)

In the *Therapeutic Communication for Health Care Professionals, 4e* MindTap platform, instructors customize the learning path by selecting Cengage Learning resources and adding their own content via apps that integrate with the MindTap framework seamlessly with many learning management systems. The guided learning path demonstrates the relevance of basic principles of therapeutic communication, through interactive quizzing and exercises, video case studies, and listening drills, elevating the study by challenging students to apply concepts to practice. To learn more, visit www.cengage.com/mindtap.

Acknowledgments

The authors and the publisher would like to thank the following reviewers for their invaluable feedback:

Lisa Graese, BA, CMT
Instructor
Spokane Community College
Spokane, WA

Tiffanie L. Hazlett, RN, BSN
Practical Nursing Instructor
Hillyard Technical Center
Saint Joseph, MO

Grant Iannelli, DC, DABCI
Adjunct Professor
DeVry University, ITT Technical Institute, Kaplan University

Carol J. Kirkner, EdD
Dean, Division of Health Sciences
Ivy Tech Community College
South Bend, IN

Christine Malone, MBA, MHA, CMPE, CPHRM, FACHE
Associate Professor and Program Director
City University of Seattle
Seattle, WA
        and
Tenured Instructor
Everett Community College
Everett, WA

David Pintado, MD, MHA, CCMA
Healthcare Program Instructor/Practicum Coordinator
Heald College
Concord, CA

Karan Serowik, RMA, CCMA
Program Director for Healthcare
Heald College
Portland, OR

David Stump-Foughty, MEd, CPC, member of AAPC
MIBC Program Director
Heald College
Portland, OR

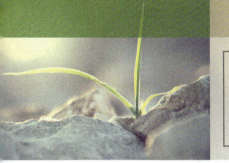

About the Authors

Carol D. Tamparo and Wilburta (Billie) Q. Lindh are coauthors of numerous health-related texts used by medical assistants and allied health care professionals throughout the United States. Both are Certified Medical Assistants, (AAMA) with more than 30 years of experience in the field and in higher education. The authors have combined education and experience at the community college, 4 year university, and graduate school levels. Their goal as educators was always to teach and model successful therapeutic communication in health care, and they continue to pursue this goal as authors.

Avenue for Feedback

Authors can be contacted at:
Carol D. Tamparo, ctamparo@comcast.net
Wilburta Q. Lindh, billie.q.l@gmail.com

Chapter 1
Therapeutic Communication

CHAPTER OBJECTIVES

After completing this chapter, the learner should be able to:

- Define key terms identified in this chapter and presented in the glossary.

- Compare professional, therapeutic, and social communications.

- List the six steps to successful professional communication.

- Summarize the various forms of social media used in the health care setting and identify goals of its use.

- Discuss the meaning of a "helping profession."

- List six questions to ask before entering a helping profession.

- Diagram the five basic elements of the communication cycle.

- Critique a minimum of four communication channels.

- Analyze the five Cs of communication and describe their effectiveness.

- Contrast verbal and nonverbal communication by using examples.

- Demonstrate nonverbal communication behaviors.

- Create a drawing to illustrate general "personal space" parameters.

- Discuss HIPAA rules for both email and fax.

- Recall at least five important points for effective team communication.

- Describe and give an example of the four selves.

Opening Case Study

An elderly woman, Mrs. Nelson, was attacked by a German shepherd while walking her toy poodle. The German shepherd came out from its yard, attacking Mrs. Nelson and her poodle on the sidewalk. Serious injuries resulted.

Mrs. Nelson was pushed onto the pavement, falling backward and striking her head. A deep, 5-inch laceration was made in the back of the skull, and heavy bleeding resulted. There were two puncture wounds in her ring finger from the dog's bite. The finger was fractured in two places. In the emergency room, she learned she also had a fractured coccyx. The toy poodle, also seriously injured, later survived emergency surgery at a veterinary clinic.

Mrs. Nelson was treated with care and compassion in an overcrowded emergency room on a Sunday night. Many health care professionals were involved in her care. Several efforts failed to stop the bleeding from the head wound, and it was several hours before Mrs. Nelson was released to go home with her finger in a splint, her head wound sutured, and a very tight bandage around her head.

She was told to see her primary care provider the next morning for a blood test to determine if there were any problems with her platelet count or in coagulation time. She was advised to return in 3 days either to the emergency room or to her doctor to have the stitches removed.

Her family called and took her to her doctor the next morning, with her emergency room records in hand.

Stop and Consider 1.1

1. Identify positive aspects of Mrs. Nelson's treatment in the emergency room.

2. You are the clinic receptionist for Mrs. Nelson's provider. What will you say to Mrs. Nelson when she arrives? What will you do for Mrs. Nelson?

The receptionist told Mrs. Nelson that she would have to wait because the doctor would not see anyone without an appointment. Mrs. Nelson explained that the emergency room provider said it was important the test be run in the morning. After more than an hour, she was finally seen and the blood test was performed.

Mrs. Nelson's provider hurriedly checked the head wound and the finger, and asked the assistant to redress the wound. Mrs. Nelson's hair was badly matted with dried blood and the assistant was uneasy about touching it. However, she did replace the bandage and sent her on her way with no instructions to return. The bandage was so loose that it fell off in the afternoon.

(continues)

Opening Case Study   (*Continued*)

Stop and Consider 1.2

1. What might Mrs. Nelson's feelings be right now?

2. Identify the positive actions in this case study.

3. Identify the negative actions in this case study.

Mrs. Nelson had hoped that her personal provider would be able to discuss her fears and anxieties, answer her questions, and give her some assurances about recovery. Mrs. Nelson's emotional needs right now were greater than her need for technical medical care. (See Maslow's Hierarchy of Needs, found in Appendix A.) When it was time to have the stitches removed, she returned to the hospital, where she felt treated with care and concern.

She was embarrassed about the dried blood in her hair, still present due to the instructions not to get the wound wet, so the nurse who helped remove the stitches used a warm washcloth and peroxide to gently remove most of the dried blood. The doctor told her the head and finger wounds were healing nicely, but that the coccyx fracture would cause her discomfort for quite some time. Mrs. Nelson left the hospital a little less traumatized, knowing it would be several weeks before she would feel like herself again.

Three months later, Mrs. Nelson needed a primary care provider's summary of her recovery process and any expected complications for insurance purposes. She returned to her primary care provider, who said, "There is nothing I can do for you now. Your head wound has healed nicely. You saw the orthopedic surgeon about your finger. I have no idea how long you will have pain from the coccyx fracture, and neither would any other provider."

Still uncomfortable about this response, she sought another provider. In her interview with the new provider, the verbal exchange turned to the accident. The provider leaned forward, seeking out the cause of Mrs. Nelson's concern, and said, "Gosh, tell me what happened." In less than 5 minutes, she poured out her story.

Recognizing Mrs. Nelson's needs, the provider asked, "How is your dog?" He also commented, "It certainly seems to me that you should be able to safely walk your dog on a public sidewalk." He then proceeded to examine her.

Technically, this final provider could do no more for the woman than either her primary care provider or the emergency room provider. What this final *provider did do, however, is listen to her, acknowledge her trauma, verify that she was not at fault, and assure her that any medical needs would be cared for to the best of his ability.*

Stop and Consider 1.3

1. Contrast the communication style of the two providers giving Mrs. Nelson care.

2. Has the first provider lost a client? Explain your response.

INTRODUCTION

This case study describes an actual ordeal, and illustrates both positive and negative communication skills. In this chapter, you are introduced to basic communication and listening skills to help you respond therapeutically to the needs of your clients. You will also become more aware of how your personal perceptions influence your personal communication style. Throughout this text you are given many examples of both therapeutic and nontherapeutic communications, reminded of the clients' right to privacy and confidentiality in the communication process, and taught how to assess your ability to be therapeutic.

THERAPEUTIC COMMUNICATION DEFINED

Professionalism

Therapeutic communication is defined as the interaction taking place between the provider and the client that is important to enhance both the physical and emotional needs of the client. It is one aspect of professionalism, which is defined as demonstrating competency and skill expected of a professional. Therapeutic communication requires clear communication of technical information in a manner that is empathetic to the client's emotional state. It requires adherence to accepted social behavior and political correctness. Therapeutic communication uses specific strategies to encourage clients to express their feelings and ideas. These expressions are then accepted by the health care professional with respect and understanding.

It includes both verbal and nonverbal communications, the language used, and how you communicate and whether you are aware of the effect you have on others. Therapeutic communication involves both professional and technical skills.

Professional Skills

Professionalism

Professional skills in the health care setting include communication, presentation, empathy, attitude, competency, integrity, and attention to detail. See Table 1-1.

TABLE 1-1   Characteristics of Health Care Professionals

Characteristics	Manifestation	Client Benefit
Communication (verbal and nonverbal)	Written communication is clear and concise and reflects clinic image Nonverbal communication reflects acceptance, values client, and expresses willingness to help	Needs are met, trust is fostered, and client is open to express health concerns
Presentation	Appears dressed and groomed appropriately Demeanor or outward behavior and conduct is respectful Expresses kindness, caring, and respect	Confident in health care choice Comfortable in setting Feels valued and respected
Empathy	Identifies with client, feels what client is feeling	Dispels fear and anxiety Comfortable
Attitude	Cultivates a positive outlook, supportive	Compliant Cooperative
Competency	Knowledgeable, skilled, competent in performing skills, dependable, demonstrates initiative, desires to continue to learn	Safe, confident, assured of confidentiality
Integrity	Honest, follows moral and ethical principles, is accountable	Builds trust, confidence, assured of confidentiality
Attention to detail	Completes correct documentation, follows all protocols of the clinic, completes all tasks	Improved health care Insurance benefits assured

You will be required to demonstrate professional skills in your interactions with clients.

Professional interaction will require you to:

1. Focus your observation.
2. Fully engage in listening.
3. Become skilled in asking open-ended questions.
4. Be intentional about affirming clients' feelings.
5. Avoid placing blame.
6. Help clients ask questions and/or express their concerns.

Becoming skilled in the six steps identified above requires another component on your part, called the "caring" component. Health care is a caring and helping profession that requires health care professionals to value and support clients.

Verbally or nonverbally, professional skills are employed every day—from the date of birth to the time of death. This communication may be a mother's soothing and loving words to a child or a simple "well done" to a colleague. Therapeutic communication focuses on enhancing the well-being of another person, and for the purposes of this text, your clients.

Technical Skills

Technical skills represent those specialized tasks that are required to deliver and support medical care. It includes skills used to explain difficult ideas and concepts, and skills to deal with difficult individuals. The opening scenario illustrates several technical skills demonstrated by the staff in the emergency room, the lab and x-ray staff support, and the assistant who bandaged the wounds. Those who assessed the injuries and followed appropriate medical-care guidelines exhibited technical skills. In comparing the responses from the two providers, one provider showed competency in technical communications but less competency in professional communication and the other was competent in *both* technical and professional communications.

PROFESSIONAL APPLICATION

As mentioned earlier, you are entering into a "helping profession." Caring must be an essential emotion for you. Are you the type of person most suited for a career in the health care profession? Some members of helping professions give so much of themselves to their clients and their work that they quickly become disillusioned and suffer burnout. Others remain so aloof and detached from their work and their clients' needs that they can become rude and disinterested. Neither situation is appropriate, successful, nor therapeutic.

Self-Awareness

Health care professionals will want to ask themselves the following simple questions:

1. *Do you genuinely enjoy helping people in a therapeutic manner?* This implies that you have the technical skills and knowledge to help people solve their problems, and that you do so without the need to create more power for yourself.

2. *Can you feel comfortable assuming a "servant" role for those in need?* "Servant" does not imply "slave," but you must genuinely enjoy serving the needs of others.

3. *Will you be able to treat any person as a "guest" no matter what their special circumstances may be?* Remember, your employment is dependent upon a satisfied customer.

4. *Can you be open to people and accept their differences?* Even though your personal lifestyle might be quite the opposite, can you be accepting and unflappable? Are you tolerant? Can you keep your opinions to yourself and be aware of your body language?

5. *Can you be firm, yet gentle?* Procedures you perform may cause discomfort and/or pain, but your verbal and nonverbal communication must convey both firmness and gentleness.

6. *Can you keep yourself out of a codependent relationship with those you help?* People in helping professions may adopt a hostile attitude toward their clients after so many years of rescuing and giving so much. Many health care professionals are harried and overcommitted, and so locked into a caretaker role that they feel dismayed and rejected when they cannot "save" someone.

Prior to considering the numerous aspects of communications more closely, read the following scenario, and ask yourself how you might respond as a health care professional. What does your response reveal about you?

Case Study: Elaine's Pregnancy Dilemma

When a young woman discovers she is pregnant, the news can be either joyous or devastating. For one young woman named Elaine, it was not good news. She was unemployed, had no money, and was very much alone. Her desperation took her to the welfare office. Elaine realized that she needed proper care for herself and the baby.

As time passed, Elaine realized that she did not have what she wanted for her baby—a place to live, two loving parents, proper medical attention, and a mother who was emotionally mature and financially secure. Elaine chose adoption as the best solution. She finally selected an adoption agency after investigating several.

After several weeks and no opportunity to identify for the agency the kind of parents Elaine would like for her baby, and little or no prenatal care assistance, she left the agency and decided to work through a private attorney for the adoption.

After only two conversations with the attorney, who explained his services for birth mothers and adoptive parents, Elaine's self-esteem improved. She completed a detailed questionnaire describing herself and her family. She completed an equally detailed summary of the kind of qualities she was looking for in parents for her baby. The attorney insisted Elaine receive prenatal care and provided her with the proper resources. Soon he matched her with a set of prospective parents.

Even though the decision had been made prior to the baby's birth about whom the adoptive parents would be, Elaine knew the final separation would be very difficult. Elaine's obstetrician and his clinic staff knew of her decision. They described for her the procedure at the hospital, and even arranged for her not to be in the maternity suite. But at no time did they discourage her from seeing her baby or deny her the rights of any other expectant mother.

At the time of the baby's delivery, the reckoning came. The comments and the nonverbal actions of the hospital staff would make the difference. Elaine was given the same treatment any other expectant mother would receive, and her best friend and birthing coach were ushered into the delivery room with her. When the baby was born, the delivery room nurse asked Elaine if she wanted to hold the baby. When Elaine said no, the nurse held her hand, smiled, and told her that was fine. She could see the baby, hold the baby, and even feed the baby at any time, if she wanted.

Stop and Consider 1.4

1. What do you think of Elaine's decision and her attitude?

2. Was the hospital staff therapeutic? Justify your response.

(continues)

Case Study   (*Continued*)

Later that day, Elaine would appear at the nursery room window, asking to see her baby. During the next 24 hours, while the attorney and adoptive parents were being notified, Elaine would hold, feed, and change this baby girl she was about to release. The adoptive parents had flown over 1,500 miles to receive the baby, so they were still a few hours away when it was time for Elaine to be discharged from the hospital.

Elaine and the adoptive parents had agreed that the baby should not go to a foster home for even a few moments, so the nurses made arrangements for Elaine to remain in the hospital, without additional charge, until the adoptive parents arrived.

The tearful exchange took place later, and Elaine gave over her daughter to be loved and cared for by the adoptive parents. One nurse assisted the ecstatic adoptive mother, while another walked the birth mother through the hospital dismissal. Elaine was deeply saddened by her loss, but she was not broken or ashamed.

Twenty-one years later, Elaine would be reunited with the daughter she allowed to be adopted. A day was spent together. They discussed similarities, including blond hair and blue eyes, their likes and dislikes—all this taking place also in the presence of the adoptive mother. At the close of the day, Elaine's daughter said, "Thanks for picking such great parents for me. I know you made a choice you thought was best for me. I love you for that and love the fact that I have two moms."

This story is repeated every day around the country. How different might it be if the comments and actions of the health care professional were critical and judgmental? Can you cite examples of both social and therapeutic communications? A closer look at how communication takes place will help assess therapeutic communications.

THE COMMUNICATION CYCLE

Communication is the sending and receiving of messages. Sometimes we are aware or conscious of the messages being sent or received and sometimes we are not. We are, however, always sending and receiving them.

Communication is a complex action in which two or more people participate. As shown in Figure 1-1, there are five basic elements involved in the communication cycle:

1. the sender,
2. the message,
3. the transmission or mode of communication,

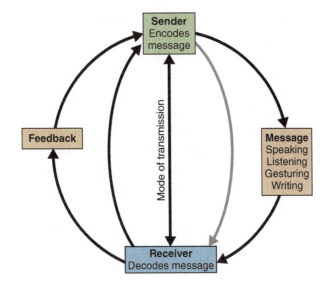

FIGURE 1-1   The communication cycle and channels of communication.

4. the receiver, and

5. feedback.

The Sender

The sender begins the communication cycle by creating or encoding the message. The sender must formulate a clear thought to send. There is great value in choosing words carefully in order to send a clear message to the receiver. Knowledge of the audience or the receiver of the particular message is important, otherwise messages can be misunderstood.

The Message

The message is the content to be communicated. The sender chooses the words and medium to best match the message to be sent. The message is most likely either spoken or in written word, but can also be categorized into verbal and nonverbal communication. The message is affected by the communication styles displayed in the sender's tone, how the message is presented, the information the message contains, and even what has been omitted.

The Transmission

How the message is actually sent is known as the transmission. This can be done through face-to-face encounters, telephone, email, texting, letters, facsimile (fax), reports, videoconferencing, and social media routes. Whatever the route, it is important to transmit the message clearly, at an appropriate time, and with the appropriate mode of transmission if the message is to be perceived correctly by the receiver. How we send and how we perceive messages, to a large extent, are based on the influences discussed earlier. Regardless of these influences, the message sent must be adapted to fit the situation and the receiver.

Each of these channels of communication has its appropriateness. In some instances, a written message may be the most effective means of communication; in other cases, spoken communication may be best. Email and videoconferencing is growing in popularity in the health care environment, and videoconferencing can be most helpful in communications involving a number of individuals or medical specialists in different areas of the country. Cell phone texting is also increasingly used in today's environment.

The Receiver

A receiver is the recipient of the sender's message. The receiver must decode the message by evaluating the communication. The primary sensory skill used in verbal communication is listening. The spoken words, as well as the tone and pitch of voice, carry meaning. Even written communications carry a "tone" that is perceived by the receiver. It may be entirely neutral, only factual, but it may also indicate care and concern by the words used and the expressions identified. Any emphasis made by the sender must be fully understood by the receiver for the message to have meaning. The receiver, however, must also remember that his or her experiences, emotions, ideas, and beliefs will enter into the sense of the message.

Feedback

Feedback occurs when the receiver and sender both verify their perception of the message. Feedback may be either verbal or nonverbal. It reveals to the sender whether the message was interpreted accurately, and enhances understanding by verifying and/or clarifying any misunderstanding. Feedback should be succinct, timely, and relevant to the situation.

VERBAL COMMUNICATION

Verbal communication refers to the sharing of information via the spoken word. Mere words, however, carry no message unless they have meaning. If you overhear a conversation in a language foreign to you, you are a witness to verbal communication, but you may not understand the message.

For communication to have any meaning, it must be understood by all parties to the communication. The book *Legal Nurse Consulting Principles* (Peterson & Kopishke, 2010) identifies the five Cs of communication. These five Cs apply equally well to therapeutic communications as well as spoken and written communication. They are (1) complete, (2) clear, (3) concise, (4) cohesive, and (5) courteous.

The message must be *complete*, with all the necessary information given. It appears that the adoption agency first told Elaine that she would be able to choose her baby's parents. What she discovered much later in the process was that she would not be able to do so until she had signed papers releasing the baby. The message was incomplete, even misleading, in its detail.

The information given in the message must also be *clear*. It must be presented in terms understandable to both parties. It is best to enunciate carefully, with good diction, to keep objects out of and away from your mouth, and to keep background noises at a minimum.

A *concise* message is one that does not include unnecessary information. Imagine how different the message would have been had the delivery room nurse said to Elaine, "Well, you really should hold this baby. She is yours. I'd certainly hold her if she were mine."

A *cohesive* message is logical and in order. It does not jump abruptly from one subject to another. You would not say to a client, "Please remove all your clothes. No, we better weigh you first. Or do you want to give us a urine sample now?" You have confused the receiver and lost his or her attention.

A message must always be *courteous* if it is to be therapeutic. Any time communication is not considerate, there is a risk that the message will be unclear, even not received, because of the defenses likely to be present in either the sender or the receiver.

NONVERBAL COMMUNICATION

Nonverbal communication is information shared without spoken words. Communicating nonverbally uses gestures and mannerisms. It is the language we learn first. It is learned seemingly automatically, as infants learn to smile in response to a smile or loving touch on the cheek long before they respond verbally.

Taber's Cyclopedic Dictionary defines body language as the unconscious use of postures, gestures, or other forms of nonverbal expression in communication. **Kinesics** is the term often used to define the systematic study of the body and the use of its static and dynamic position as a means of communication.

Cultural

⊕ Much of our body language is a learned behavior and is greatly influenced by the culture in which we are raised. For example, eye contact may send different nonverbal messages depending on the culture of the client. These variations make it important to assess clients' cultural identity to ensure proper nonverbal communication.

Feelings are communicated quite well nonverbally. Since nonverbal communication is much less subject to conscious control, emotional dimensions are often expressed nonverbally. The body naturally expresses our true, repressed feelings. Most of the negative messages we express nonverbally are unintended. But whether they are intentional or not, the message is relayed. Experts tell us that 70% of communication is nonverbal. The tone of voice communicates 23% of the message, and only 7% of the message is actually communicated in what is said.

Two Key Points to Successful Nonverbal Communication

There are two key points to remember in any successful communication.

- First, there must be congruency between the verbal and the nonverbal expressed message. This means the two messages must be in agreement or be consistent with each other. If I verbally tell you I am not angry, but speak in angry tones and have my fists clenched and my face contorted, I am sending a mixed message. Chances are you will believe my nonverbal message rather than the verbal.
- Second, remember that nonverbal cues appear in groups. The grouping of gestures, facial expressions, and postures into nonverbal statements is known as **clustering**. In the previous example, the tone of voice, the gesture of clenched fists, and the facial expression form a nonverbal statement or cluster of cues to true feelings and emotions.

TYPES OF NONVERBAL COMMUNICATION

Facial Expression

Eye contact is another form of facial expression, and is often viewed as a sign of interest in the individual. It provides cues to indicate that what others say is important. A long stare may be interpreted as an invasion of privacy, which creates an uncomfortable, uneasy feeling. A lack of eye contact in

Western culture is usually interpreted to mean a lack of involvement, or avoidance.

Perhaps the most important nonverbal communicator is facial expression. It has been said that the eyes mirror the soul. Certain movements of the eyebrow seem to indicate questioning, while others may disclose feelings of amusement, surprise, puzzlement, or worry. The manner in which the forehead is wrinkled also sends similar messages. The eyes can communicate several kinds of messages. Have you ever seen laughter and joy, grief, or pain reflected in another's eyes?

Touch

Touch is one of the most sensitive means of communication. Touch is often used to express deep feelings that are impossible to express verbally, and can be a very powerful means of communication.

For all health care professionals, many tasks involve touching the client. Most clients will understand and accept the touching behavior, as it is related to the medical setting. Some clients, however, are not comfortable being touched, so sensitivity is essential. It is helpful to tell clients when, where, and how they are to be touched during an examination. Explaining all assessments and treatments tends to put individuals at ease. This technique is essential when a client is autistic. An individual with autism has heightened sensory abilities and may attempt to escape sensory overload or a sudden invasion of their personal space. They tend to want to get away from strange people, voices, and equipment. If you find yourself in a helping situation or profession and feel uncomfortable touching, self-assessment or self-awareness may be necessary.

Touch is often synonymous with reassurance, understanding, and caring. It is important to assess our level of comfort, and that of the client, in relation to the use of touch. When we are comfortable using touch and when we are sensitive to a client's level of acceptance to touch, touch can be used in a therapeutic manner.

Personal Space

Personal space is the distance at which individuals are comfortable with others. It may be determined by social and cultural influences. Personal space can be thought of as the invisible fence no one can see. However, the *way* in which we define boundaries *is* evident to others.

Cultural

⊕ We feel threatened when others invade our personal space without our consent. Many individuals have well-defined personal space boundaries.

Examples of personal space in Western culture are listed below for your consideration.

Intimate	—	touching to 1½ feet
Personal	—	1½–4 feet
Social	—	4–12 feet (most often observed)
Public	—	12–15 feet

Many cultures uphold these four categories of spatial relationships; however, the distances may vary from one culture to another.

Many medically related tasks involve invading another's personal space. It is beneficial to explain procedures that intrude on another's space before beginning the procedure. This gives the client some control and a sense of dignity and worth.

Position

When speaking with a client, it is helpful to maintain a close but comfortable position. Standing over a client denotes superiority, while too much distance may be interpreted as being exclusive or avoiding. Movement toward a client usually indicates warmth, liking, interest, acceptance, and trust. Moving away may suggest dislike, disinterest, boredom, indifference, suspicion, or impatience (see Figure 1-2).

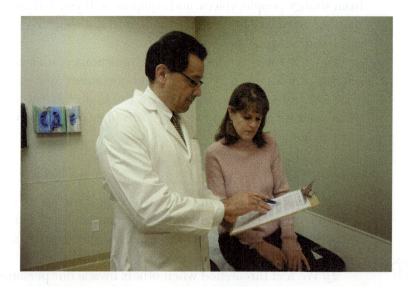

FIGURE 1-2   Positive posture and position encourage therapeutic communication.

Posture

Like distance, posture is important to the health care professional. Individuals in threatening situations usually tense, but tend to relax in a nonthreatening environment. Posture can be used as a barometer for feelings. For example, sitting with the limbs crossed over one's chest can send a message of closure and avoidance; leaning back in a chair with the arms up and hands clasped behind the head can indicate openness to suggestions.

Slumped shoulders may signal depression, discouragement, or in some cases even pain. It is important to validate the messages before continuing a procedure. For example, you may ask the client, "Are you comfortable?" or "Is this position too painful?" Technicians must be careful to be in tune with the client's physical comfort.

Gestures/Mannerisms

Most everyone uses gestures or "talks" with their hands to some degree. Gestures are useful in emphasizing ideas, in creating and holding others' attention, and in relieving stress. Some common gestures and their perceived meanings might be:

Finger-tapping	—	impatience, nervousness, rudeness
Shrugged shoulders	—	indifference, discouragement
Rubbing the nose	—	puzzlement
Whitened knuckles and clenched fists	—	anger
Fidgeting	—	nervousness, anxiety

It is important to recognize that nonverbal communication helps understanding, and frequently is more powerful than verbal communication. It is also more enduring and has more persuasive power than verbal communication. The nonverbal message is more quickly believed than the verbal message.

WORD OF CAUTION

It must be remembered, however, that nonverbal communication can easily be misinterpreted. The folded arms may mean the person is cold, not closed to communication. The wrinkled brow may indicate the person has a headache, not a questioning or doubting attitude. Look for congruency between verbal and nonverbal communication for a clear message. Do not make assumptions.

In the earlier scenario, when the delivery room nurse asked Elaine if she would like to hold the baby, the verbal and nonverbal messages were congruent. When Elaine said no, the nurse held her hand, smiled, and told her that was fine. Together, the cluster of mannerisms used by the delivery room nurse said, "I understand, I care, and your response is appropriate."

LISTENING SKILLS

Listening is often identified as the passive aspect of communication. However, if done well, listening is very active. Good listeners have their eyes upon the speaker, are attentive, and are aware of the nonverbal messages as well as the verbal information coming from the sender. Effective listening requires concentration.

Therapeutic listening includes listening with a "third ear": that is, being aware of what the client is *not* saying or picking up on hints as to the real message. In the scenario of Mrs. Nelson at the beginning of this chapter, her primary care provider (PCP) was either unaware of the nonverbal cues and hints being made or chose to see them as unimportant.

The health care professional should have three listening goals: (1) to improve listening skills sufficiently so that clients are heard accurately; (2) to listen for what is not being said or for information transmitted only by hints; and (3) to determine how accurately the message has been received.

A technique used by many and suggested by professionals is the ability to paraphrase the client's message or statement. This technique allows the receiver of the message to return the message to the sender, perhaps worded differently, allowing the sender to acknowledge the accuracy of the message.

Sender: "Will I be able to use my medical coupons for prenatal care in your clinic?"

Receiver: "You're concerned about whether our doctor accepts medical coupons for payment."

Sender: "That's correct. I have no money. My baby will be adopted, but I know we both need proper medical care."

Receiver: "Our clinic does take medical coupons, and we make no distinction in our care whether you pay privately or use your coupon. Would you like to make an appointment?"

This example shows both active listening and therapeutic communication skills. The clinic assistant heard both concerns—the monetary concern and the concern for quality and proper care.

Health care professionals must be prudent in how they use active listening techniques, however. It is not appropriate to paraphrase everything the client says; otherwise, the client begins to feel stupid, or believes the professional has a hearing problem.

One of the greatest barriers to listening occurs when receivers find themselves thinking about something else while trying to listen. It is difficult to try to concentrate on what is being said when the mind is wandering. When this happens, pull concentration back to the sender, apologize if necessary, and continue with the communication.

There is a time in communication, in listening, when silence is appropriate. So many times health care professionals try to "fix" everything with a recommendation, a prescription, or even advice. Sometimes none of those things are necessary. The client simply needs someone to listen, to acknowledge the difficulty, and to remember that the client is not helpless in finding a solution to the problem.

Skill in communication takes years of practice and frequent review. It will never become perfect; the goal is to become *better* at it with each passing day. Communication is and always will be the very basis for any therapeutic relationship.

INFLUENCE OF TECHNOLOGY ON COMMUNICATION

There will always be face-to-face communication, telephone conversations between two individuals, and paper communication in the health care setting, but email, fax, text messaging, and video and teleconferencing are increasingly common in health care. Personal electronic devices such as smartphones, tablets, and laptop computers can be linked to a network for Internet access or communication with satellite facilities from almost anywhere in the world. In this environment, however, the content of the message is most likely to be examined for credibility without any of the nonverbal cues such as eye contact, facial expression, or posture. Communication interactions when using this technology require careful consideration.

The use of *email* is popular in the health care setting, both in communication with clients and in communication with colleagues. It may be read at the convenience of the receiver. Clients are particularly interested in the use of email for such things as prescription refills, appointment scheduling, information updates, or simple requests that normally would not require a visit and are more convenient than placing a telephone call, leaving a message, and waiting for a response.

Email communication is used only for clients who have been examined within the last 6 months. No information can be provided through email without the clients' release of information to do so. Only clients can determine what, if any, personal health information (PHI) can be shared.

Legal

 The **Health Insurance Portability and Accountability Act (HIPAA)** is very specific in its guidelines for electronic transmission of client information. It is not the purpose of this text to detail HIPAA guidelines, but the Web site for the Department of Health and Human Services is helpful (www.hhs.gov).

General guidelines for all email etiquette include the following:

- Be concise and to the point.
- Respond in a timely fashion and answer all questions.
- Use proper spelling and grammar.
- Do not attach unnecessary files.
- Do not write in CAPITALS.
- Add disclaimers to the email.
- Read any email carefully before pressing "Send."
- Any clinical email regarding a client should be copied and placed in the medical record.

Fax messaging uses telephone lines to transmit data from one fax machine to another. It is often used for referrals, insurance approvals, and informal correspondence. The same standards of confidentiality for any client information identified in an email exist for fax communication. HIPAA requirements dictate that fax machines are not to be placed in a centralized area where unauthorized individuals may see documents being sent by fax. A cover sheet should be included that stipulates the information is for the intended recipient only. Fax messaging saves the time and effort of copying and mailing a document, allowing the sender to keep the original while providing the recipient with an exact duplicate.

Satellite *video* and *teleconferencing* are used to share information, receive education and training in a particular field of health care, or conduct a meeting to make certain decisions. A video conference will allow participants to see one another and interact almost as if the individuals were together in one room. A teleconference consists of a group of individuals connected by only a telephone. Both video and teleconferences can become difficult to manage if more than 10 participants are included. A telephone conference should be limited to 30 minutes or less, since it is difficult for participants to concentrate while looking into space for any longer period of time.

Effective video and teleconferencing, as well as telephone conference calls, include some basic rules of conduct:

- One person is the facilitator and is responsible for keeping the meeting on track.
- Come prepared with necessary documents or information that is to be shared.
- Before speaking, remember that everyone may not recognize your voice or know who you are; always begin with "This is _____."
- Silence is not bad. Facial expressions may not be evident, and someone may be formulating a question prior to speaking. Also, do not assume silence means consent.
- Stay focused on the meeting. The conscious mind cannot perform some other task and give full attention to the meeting at the same time.

SOCIAL MEDIA IN HEALTH CARE

In today's society, many individuals communicate via **social media**. Social media can be used for education, obtaining information, networking, goal setting, receiving support (i.e., losing weight or lowering blood sugar levels), and tracking personal progress. Health care providers increasingly turn toward online social media to connect with clients and share information about particular issues in health care or share the latest news of the clinic. Facebook, Twitter, and YouTube are most commonly used. For example, a PCP might send a message to remind everyone to get a flu shot. A pediatrician might use a **blog** to share information with clients who have diabetes and who then can connect with others with similar needs. A quick Internet search reveals many different social media sites for almost any health condition and group of people. For instance, breastcancer.org provides an online community for those diagnosed with breast cancer, including informational pages and newsletters, blogs, discussion boards, and podcasts.

Client-centered care is one of the primary goals of social media used within the health care environment. Increasingly, clients prefer social media for setting appointments and receiving reminders, getting test results, refilling prescriptions, and getting answers to general questions. Twitter is often used to connect with other professionals about specific topics of interest to providers. The National Institutes of Health reports that PCPs use social media to read news articles, explore the latest drug research, and communicate with other providers regarding health care issues.

TEAM COMMUNICATION

Effective communication is essential to effective team interactions in the workplace. It is helpful if health care professionals receive specialized training in the facility's protocol for the use and dissemination of all forms of communications. Not only is there emphasis upon communication with clients and customers, the same attention is to be paid to communication among employees and providers. A sensitive employee can easily determine if another employee or one of the providers is having a "not so good" day. A warm greeting, the offer of a cup of coffee, a friendly gesture—all these go a long way in turning that day into something better for everyone in terms of productivity and accomplishments. All the guidelines and recommendations in this chapter are to be employed in team communication to help make the facility run more smoothly. Remember, your clients are smart. They will immediately pick up the vibes of discontent from employees when it exists.

Effective communicators in the health care team will strive to do the following:

- Listen carefully to others.
- Explain their ideas clearly.
- Clarify others' ideas as necessary.
- Express feelings in a nonthreatening manner.
- Check for feelings based on nonverbal cues.
- Initiate conversations with others if there appears to be tension.
- Encourage others to be effective communicators.

There also must be guidelines or policies on what can be communicated via email and any social media used within the facility and among coworkers. Some simple rules to consider follow:

- Do not use email if a walk into an adjacent office for a face-to-face communication is possible.
- Reserve two to four times daily to check email; notify others of your decision. Otherwise, you can become a "slave" to the technology.

- Answer email within a 24-hour time period.
- Create a response message when you are out of the facility for any period of time.
- Remember that email is not private.
- Be careful what you forward and seek permission when you do so.
- Do not use the facility's computer for personal email or any form of social media.
- Use "flags" and "Important" sparingly.
- Never send libelous, defamatory, offensive, racist, or obscene remarks.

In order to communicate effectively as a team member, take time to develop skills that will ensure trust, and to build into the team a sense of worth and importance.

Successful team communication requires collaboration. That means that health care professionals assume complementary roles and work together in a cooperative manner. Responsibilities are shared because there is an awareness of each other's knowledge, skills, education, and training. There is also a shared goal of carrying out plans for clients' care and working together for a common goal or common aim. Such an interdisciplinary approach pools the specialized services of each team member into an individualized care program for each client. Clients will find it more comfortable to communicate with a cohesive team rather than with individuals who do not know what others are doing in the client's care.

Stop and Consider 1.5

You are in a conversation with a professional regarding data usage on your cell phone. It appears that you are losing data that you actually have not used. After much checking by the professional and your responses to questions asked, the professional admits that a supervisor needs to be involved. You are transferred to a supervisor who can hopefully solve the problem. When the supervisor comes on the line, you have to explain the situation all over again because this individual knows nothing about your issue.

1. How do you feel about the cell phone service?

2. What is missing in this team's communication?

3. What might have occurred to make this professional and technical communication cohesive and therapeutic?

LIFE FACTORS THAT INFLUENCE COMMUNICATIONS

How you feel about yourself can and will directly affect how therapeutic you will be in both social and professional communications. There are a number of factors that influence your personal communication skills. They are neither good nor bad; they simply are a part of your heritage, culture, and lifestyle. These factors greatly impact our lives and dominate how we feel about ourselves and how we feel others perceive us. A few of these factors are listed here.

Genetic Factors

Inherited traits, such as height, body structure, and skin color, are defined and established by the genes passed on during fertilization. Even our gender influences perception. Nurses in hospital nurseries will tell you that every infant born has a unique personality. This is because even our personalities have a genetic component. Personality traits are **polygenic**, meaning multiple genes are involved in determining a trait that is then manipulated by life experiences.

Cultural Factors

Cultural

⊕ Every culture has its own customs and traditions that directly influence the person we are and how we are perceived. For example, in Western medical tradition, we look directly at someone when speaking and often address individuals using first names. In many cultures, however, it is disrespectful to look directly at another person (especially one in authority), or to use first names when addressing them. This topic is discussed more fully in Chapter 2, "Multicultural Therapeutic Communication."

Economic Factors

A person's financial status often relates directly to the type of education and life experiences they possess. If you were born and raised in poverty, your perception of life and others is likely to be much different than if you were born and raised in affluence. The amount and type of education and job training experience is a direct influence on perception.

Life Experiences

Life experiences are great teachers. Those who have experienced grief and loss generally respond with a deeper sensitivity to others than do those who have not experienced grief and loss. Whether life's trials have been fairly easy or very harsh will influence one's lifestyle.

Spiritual and Moral Values

Spiritual beliefs influence perception. A spiritual belief in one's life can influence an individual's attitude when caring for others' needs. Spirituality generally encourages a reach beyond the self to guide and care for others. Values or morals, the rules we live by or habits of conduct, are important in relation to self and others. This fact can make it difficult to relate to someone with entirely different rules of conduct or habits that you follow.

Role Models

Role models are found in national leaders, parents, teachers, spiritual guides, and public figures. They can be either positive or negative, but are likely to have a powerful influence over a long period of time. Positive role models can help cultivate sensitivity, confidence, and social skills. Negative role models can either channel one's desires toward creating more positive actions or more deeply reinforce the negative actions.

SELF-AWARENESS AND THE THERAPEUTIC PROCESS

Self-Awareness

To begin the therapeutic process, we must learn to recognize and evaluate our own actions and responses in given situations. It is important to know how we feel, understand, and like ourselves before we can begin to understand and like others.

What Is Self-Awareness?

Self-awareness is being aware of oneself as an individual. It includes all the beliefs a person has with respect to behavior. It is the mental image of the self, and may be realistic or unrealistic. Self-awareness begins to form at a very early age and is well established by the age of 6. It is also changeable, however, and is affected by all the influences mentioned earlier and many more.

Before going further, take time now to complete the "I am" statements in Exercise 1 in this chapter. This exercise will stimulate your thinking about yourself and assist you in making some assessments about yourself as well. Do you accept yourself as you are now, or would you like to make some changes? Would you add any "I am" statements?

While we cannot do much to change many of the things that influence our lives, we *can* recognize their presence, evaluate their effect, and begin to initiate changes as necessary. One way to do this is through self-assessment.

The Value of Self-Assessment

The value of *self-assessment* is that it helps us determine who we are, as seen by the self and by others. It is a tool to illustrate both positive and negative characteristics so that changes may be implemented. These changes encourage growth and keep us from becoming stagnant. Self-assessment gives us the power to accept or alter these changes.

Each of us has at least three selves: the *ideal self*, the *public self*, and the *real self*. The *ideal self* is the person we think we should be and the person we would like to become. The *public self* is how we want others to see us. We may have many public selves, depending upon the circle of people with whom we have contact. The public self is our reputation. The *real self* is the inner, natural self, authentic, and spontaneous. When you are most true to yourself and transparent to others, you are being your real self.

Some psychologists identify a fourth self called the *critic self*. This is the inner "shaming" voice. Shame, or the feeling we do not meet others' expectations of us, may start in childhood and be passed from generation to generation. Shame occurs in families where secrets are kept about addiction, infidelity, or anything that is kept quiet in order to keep up appearances. Teachers may shame students who do not perform well in their studies. Others may shame you for expressing anger or sadness. Shame can camouflage the *real self*, allowing the *critic self* to suppress the *real self*.

In order to have positive self-acceptance, there must be a congruency between the three selves and the critic self must be well understood and not allowed to undermine the real self. There should be balance and a good feeling about each dimension.

Complete Exercise 2, which is related to the four selves, to assist you in determining how you personally feel about these dimensions of yourself. What did you learn about yourself? Can you make any changes in your life to facilitate growth?

SUMMARY

Understanding self and the basic components of communication is vital to establishing a therapeutic relationship with clients, who likely come to the "helping relationship" with a number of barriers that impede communication. Clients may be anxious, experiencing pain, or be very ill. Communication that understands these barriers, keeps in mind the communication cycle, and comes from health care professionals who know and understand themselves will help empower clients to be full participants in the client–professional relationship. Remember, too, that effective communication skills require special attention when interacting with others when nonverbal cues cannot be assessed, such as in email or social media. Recall the statement made earlier regarding confidentiality and not entering into any media form of communication without specific agreements with clients. With that step in place, most of the media sites are able to support HIPAA-compliant one-on-one messages and discussion forums. As with any other communication, recall the five Cs of communication when engaged in social media communications. In all communications, either within the clinic environment or with clients, strive for a pattern of openness, trust, support, and respect.

EXERCISES

Exercise 1

Read the following statements and select the 10 statements you think best describe you. Then select 10 statements you think *least* describe you. Ask a friend to indicate the statements they think describe you the best, and the least.

"I AM" STATEMENTS

I am a perfectionist.	I am afraid of failure.
I am dependable.	I am hard to get along with.
I am reserved.	I am competitive.
I am realistic.	I am ambitious.
I am a happy person.	I am courageous.
I am well liked.	I am an understanding person.
I am easily hurt.	I am often depressed.
I am impulsive.	I am easygoing.
I am self-conscious.	I am socially adept.
I am secure.	I am often lonely.
I am sympathetic.	I am in control.
I am able to express emotions.	I am socially inept.
I am unpredictable.	I am disorganized.
I am often opinionated.	I am well groomed.
I am creative.	I am attractive.
I am self-reliant.	I am selfish.
I am naive.	I am a decision maker.
I am sometimes incompetent.	I am unattractive.

I am self-sacrificing.

I am generous.

I am able to live by rules.

I am a worrier.

I am shy.

I am intelligent.

I have a good self-image.

I am a people person.

I am assertive.

I am fickle.

I am argumentative.

I am fun-loving.

I am often suspicious of others.

I am confident.

I am precise.

I am realistic.

I am overprotective.

I am energetic.

I am tolerant.

I am responsible for myself.

I am content.

I am often insecure.

I am generally trusting.

I am usually able to make decisions.

I am oversensitive.

I am poised.

Exercise 2

Using the columns provided, list adjectives that describe how you might perceive yourself.

Ideal Self	Public Self	Real Self	Critic Self
Ask the question, "What kind of person do I wish to become?"	You may wish to ask someone who knows you to describe you.	What do you really feel inside?	Do I feel shame? If so, when, how?

Exercise 3

Write a paragraph discussing a recent incident, preferably personal, in which a communicator failed to communicate what was intended. Analyze why this happened and how it could have been avoided.

REVIEW QUESTIONS

Multiple Choice

1. How are technical skills best described?

   a. Specific and specialized tasks are required.

   b. They are only necessary in the health care setting.

   c. They are interpersonal skills both in professional and personal relationships.

   d. They are not exhibited through nonverbal communication.

2. Which of the following is true about therapeutic communication?

   a. Specific and well-defined professional skills are required.

   b. There is no influence by personal feelings of self.

   c. It takes place only in verbal communication.

   d. It does not change with culture.

3. Can you list the four selves?

   a. Social self, real self, hidden self, and critic self

   b. Ideal self, critic self, hidden self, and public self

   c. Critic self, social self, ideal self, and real self

   d. Ideal self, public self, real self, and critic self

4. What is essential in the feedback element of the communication cycle?

   a. The message is encoded and verified.

   b. The message will always be verbal in format.

   c. The receiver gets the message, decodes it, and verifies it with the sender.

   d. Speaking, listening, gesturing, and writing form the elements of feedback.

5. What are the five Cs of verbal communication?

   a. Complete, clear, concise, courteous, congruent

   b. Complete, clear, concise, cohesive, courteous

   c. Correct, concise, concrete, complete, courteous

   d. Correct, clear, complete, courteous, congruent

6. According to experts, what percentage of communication is nonverbal?

   a. 32%   **c.** 70%

   b. 7%   **d.** 93%

7. Which of the following best defines effective listening?

   a. It is the passive part of communication, making it unimportant.

   b. It requires concentration and is very active.

   c. It comes naturally to most individuals and is the easiest part of communication.

   d. It pays attention only to the spoken word.

8. Communication using electronic media does not easily evaluate which of the following?

   a. Cultural diversity   **c.** Listening skills

   b. Nonverbal cues   **d.** Content credibility

9. In the opening case study, the nurse says, "Mrs. Nelson, I believe I can get most of the dried blood from your hair with a warm cloth and some peroxide if you have just a little bit of time." What kind of skill is being demonstrated?

   a. Social communication skills   **c.** Technical relations skills

           d. Professional communication skills

   b. Human relations skills

10. Two clients are being seen in the clinic by different providers at the same time. They have checked in and their addresses, telephone numbers, and insurance status were identified. One client has the state's new insurance under the National Health Care Plan; the other client has a comprehensive health care plan provided by the communities' largest employer. What factor is in place here?

   a. Genetic factors   **c.** Life experiences

   b. Economic factors   **d.** Moral values

FOR FURTHER CONSIDERATION

1. On a sheet of paper, identify and describe yourself as briefly and as fully as possible. (For instance, I am a woman, a mother, a grand-mother; I am Native American; I am a sister to four siblings; etc.) For each descriptive, explain how to relate to an individual who is just the opposite, or quite different. (For instance, a man, a father, a grandfa-ther, or someone who is not a parent; a man from East India; an only child; etc.) How do you communicate professionally and therapeuti-cally, realizing these differences?

2. Go to the section in this chapter on Professional Application on p. 7 and respond to question 3. Identify how you might be able to treat someone as a "guest" in a health care setting when he or she is someone you would not have as a guest in your home. List the rea-sons why this individual would *not* be a guest in your home. What do you do to remain therapeutic? Do you have any prejudices to reconsider?

3. Can you be sympathetic with Elaine in the case study "Elaine's Pregnancy Dilemma"? Could you place your newborn for adoption? If not, and you are the health care professional assigned to Elaine during delivery, what will you do to communicate therapeutically?

4. Now that you have finished this chapter, will there be any changes you will make personally in the way you communicate either socially or professionally? If so, identify the changes you will make.

CASE STUDIES

Case Study 1

Zena is a home health care aide. She is assisting an 83-year-old woman to dress herself when the woman stumbles and slumps to the floor. As Zena gets down to help her, the woman begins to cry and says, "I am so useless; I can't do anything anymore." What should Zena do? What might Zena say?

Case Study 2

You are a receptionist in a skilled nursing facility. You are expecting a new resident this afternoon. He is an 85-year-old gentleman who is coming for several days of rehabilitation prior to release to his home. His wife, age 82, is awaiting hip replacement surgery and walks with a cane. You happen to look out the glass door to see a taxi pull up. You see that this is your new admit and his wife. The taxi driver does not get out of the car or open the door for his passengers. You observe their struggle to exit the taxi.

1. What are the passengers feeling at this point?

2. What will you do?

3. What kinds of skills will you demonstrate?

REFERENCES AND RESOURCES

Antai-Otong, D. (2007). *Psychiatric nursing: Biological and behavioral concepts*. Clifton Park, NY: Cengage Learning.

Connected Living, Inc. (2013). Senior living technology. Retrieved from www.connectedliving.com.

Hosley, J., & Molle, E. (2006). *A practical guide to therapeutic communication for health professionals*. St Louis, MO: Saunders Elsevier.

Househ, M. (2013). The use of social media in healthcare: Organizational, clinical, and patient perspectives. *Studies in Health Technology and Informatics*, 183, 244–248.

Lindh, W. Q., Pooler, M., Tamparo, C. D., Dahl, B., & Morris, J. (2014). *Administrative medical assisting* (5th ed.). Clifton Park, NY: Cengage Learning.

Peterson, A. M., & Kopishke, L. (Eds.). (2010). *Legal nurse consulting principles* (3rd ed.). Boca Raton, FL: CRC Press.

Silverman, J., Kurtz, S., Draper, J., Deveuele, M., & Suchman, A. L. (2013). *Skills for communicating with patients* (3rd ed.). London: Radcliffe.

Venes, D. (2013). *Taber's cyclopedic medical dictionary* (22nd ed.). Philadelphia: F.A. Davis.

Chapter 2
Multicultural Therapeutic Communication

CHAPTER OBJECTIVES

After completing this chapter, the learner should be able to:

- Define key terms as presented in the glossary.

- Recall three important actions to promote multicultural communication.

- Analyze the eight barriers to multicultural communication listed in this chapter.

- Describe practical ways to personally begin to understand and implement therapeutic multicultural communication.

- Distinguish between bias, prejudice, and ethnocentrism, and identify common biases and prejudices that may be experienced in today's health care facilities.

- Describe characteristics of low- and high-context communication styles.

- Summarize the caregiving structure of various cultures.

- Recall the socioeconomic environment of individuals and cultures regarding time focus.

- Describe Maslow's Hierarchy of Needs and its relationship to time focus.

- Contrast how culture and religion impact attitudes relating to health care and therapeutic communication.

- Identify several accommodations providers could consider for multicultural clients and those with language and hearing loss or speech impairment.

- Summarize the benefits of using a medical interpreter and the guidelines to follow when working with a medical interpreter.

- Apply therapeutic techniques when interacting with multicultural clients and those with language and hearing or speech impairment.

Opening Case Study

Beatrice completed her medical assistant education near her hometown in rural Wisconsin and, because of better opportunities for employment, moved to Newark, New Jersey, to follow her career goal of becoming a physician assistant. She was hired as an MA in a clinic in a predominantly middle-class, working neighborhood populated primarily by families who are Puerto Rican and African American. While Beatrice was preparing a client for examination, the client said she thought her previous doctor was very "bad." Beatrice was shocked and did not know what to say or do about this statement.

Stop and Consider 2.1

1. What do you think the client means by the statement "my previous doctor was very bad"?

2. What response would you make?

INTRODUCTION

Cultural

⊕ The opening case study illustrates a communication challenge directly related to cultural differences between the client and the health care professional. Cultural differences may exist in many ways, including language, dress, nonverbal cues, and body structure. The population of the United States is one of the most ethnically and culturally diverse countries in the world. Not only do we see more cultural diversity in our clients, but we also experience clinicians from a variety of cultural backgrounds to further challenge communication.

Recall from Chapter 1 that only 7% of the meaning and intent of communication is based on the actual words spoken. Words should be chosen very carefully and nonverbal cues that may hinder therapeutic communication should be avoided. Understanding that some cultures ascribe specific meaning to eye contact, some facial expressions, touch, tone of voice, and nods of the head will be helpful.

Successfully achieving multicultural therapeutic communication requires consideration of the cultural background of the client. According to the 2010 Census, slightly more than one-third of the population of the United States comes from a culture other than American (i.e., Caucasian English-speaking Judeo-Christian) (Humes, Jones, & Ramirez, 2011). See Figure 2-1.

The United States is also sexually diverse. Lesbian, gay, bisexual, and transgender (LGBT) persons constitute 3.8% of the overall population. This is an important distinction because based on a 2013 National Health Interview Survey, LGBT clients will have more health-related issues than heterosexual clients (Ward, Dahlhamer, Galinsky, & Joestl, 2014). Consequently, the number of LGBT clients is likely to be greater than indicated by the survey. Therapeutic communication with LGBT clients will involve all of the challenges encountered with clients of other cultures and religions, but with one additional challenge: the greater likelihood of bias or prejudice on the

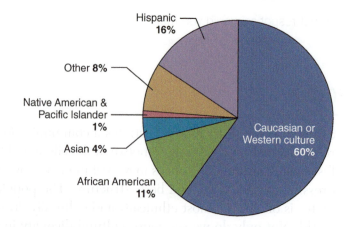

FIGURE 2-1   United States Demographic Makeup (2010 Census).
Source: United States Census 2010.

part of health care professionals. According to a May 2013 Pew Research Center survey, 39% of those surveyed showed a negative bias toward the LGBT community. This bias and prejudice is not limited to only LGBT clients, the same survey showed a negative bias against people who are Muslim (45%), Hispanic (25%), and African American (22%). As a health care professional, it is important to identify your biases and prejudices and take steps to eliminate them.

Some of the predominant ethnic/religious cultural characteristics that may affect therapeutic communication are discussed in this chapter. In this text, the authors generalize similar cultures together to establish a knowledge base to be used in understanding clients of ethnic diversity. Medical professionals working within a specific cultural community will want to seek further information relating to that particular culture or individual client. In many instances, health care professionals can develop rapport with their ethnically diverse clients by simply demonstrating an interest in their culture and background.

DEVELOPING MULTICULTURAL COMMUNICATION

A **culture** is a way of life of a group of people—the behaviors, beliefs, values, and symbols that they accept, generally without thinking about them, and that are passed along by communication and imitation from one generation to the next.

Self-Awareness

Multicultural communication is the ability to communicate effectively with individuals of other cultures while recognizing one's own personal cultural biases and prejudices and putting them aside. Such recognition requires being aware of the differences and likenesses among human beings and willingly accepting the uniqueness of each other. Three important actions to promote multicultural communication are (1) to become knowledgeable about the beliefs and values of different cultures, (2) to recognize barriers to multicultural communication, and (3) to develop techniques that build and foster multicultural communication.

Therapeutic communication takes place between an individual who has a specific need, no matter what his or her culture, lifestyle, or religious status is, and a person who is skilled in techniques that can identify, resolve, or satisfy that need. Therapeutic communication is goal-oriented. When health care professionals engage in multicultural therapeutic communication, clients from different cultures, lifestyles, and religions are assisted with their health-related goals.

BARRIERS TO MULTICULTURAL THERAPEUTIC COMMUNICATION

In her book *Transcultural Communication in Health Care*, Joan Luckmann (2000) identifies eight barriers to therapeutic transcultural communication: (1) lack of knowledge; (2) fear and distrust; (3) racism; (4) bias, prejudice, and ethnocentrism; (5) stereotyping; (6) health care rituals; (7) language; and (8) differences in perceptions and expectations. The following paragraphs explore each of these barriers and discuss tactics for overcoming or diminishing them within health care settings.

Lack of Knowledge

In order to provide culturally sensitive health care, health care professionals must understand and take into consideration the cultural differences of their clients. The first step is to learn more about clients' cultures. Begin by making a list of the cultures served in your clinic and conduct a systematic study of each. Libraries contain autobiographies, biographies, novels, and essays related to various cultures. The Internet is another useful resource. Television provides travel documentary programs that are both interesting and informative. Enjoy a restaurant meal with a different cultural cuisine. Consider involving staff in a culture-of-the-month study. At the end of the month, an in-house luncheon could be shared, with each staff member bringing a food contribution representing the month's culture. Sharing the knowledge learned broadens the base for each staff member and builds a comfort level for interacting with clients of other cultures.

Fear and Distrust

Both the provider and client may experience fear during a multicultural exchange. When meeting someone from another culture, one's first response or reaction may be reservation because the other person looks, dresses, or smells different, or may communicate in a language or **dialect** that you may not understand. In the health care setting, the client is in unfamiliar surroundings and is in a subordinate position to the provider. Under these conditions a reserved attitude can become fear or concern because of a lack of understanding of the culture. Confusion from the messages being sent, verbally and nonverbally, may lead to feelings of dislike and distrust. Knowing more about the other culture helps to dispel these emotions. When the cause of this fear and distrust is recognized, cross-cultural communication becomes easier.

Racism

Race includes any of the major biological divisions of mankind, distinguished by, for example, skin or eye color, hair texture, stature, or body proportions. Racism implies racial discrimination, segregation, persecution, and domination. Individuals, cultural groups, or institutions can experience racism. Most everyone has some racial biases toward one or more cultures or races. Often this bias or prejudice is based on hearsay or not understanding the culture. Actual racism or perceived racism results in fear and distrust between client and health care provider, with a resulting negative impact on therapeutic communication. It is beyond the scope of this text to resolve the problem, but it is possible to highlight what individuals can do to become more racially tolerant.

The elimination of racism in an individual begins with knowledge and the examination of conscious and unconscious attitudes regarding race and culture. The next step is a commitment to changing the attitude(s). Engaging in open and honest discussions with others helps in recognizing personal feelings on the subject and reinforces a commitment to eliminate racism.

Bias, Prejudice, and Ethnocentrism

Self-Awareness

Bias is a slant toward a particular belief. Synonyms for bias may include favoritism, one-sidedness, trend, inclination, or feeling. Bias may indicate that you are in favor of or against something, usually in a way considered to be unfair. **Prejudice** is an opinion or judgment that is formed before all of the facts are known; prejudice is usually preconceived and unfavorable. Most prejudices are learned socially and are often based on misconception and misunderstanding. Body language may also unconsciously transmit bias or prejudice.

Ethnocentrism is the belief that one's own culture and traditions are better than those of another. An example of ethnocentrism would be to refuse to bow to greet a Japanese acquaintance or associate and to insist on shaking hands. Health care professionals must be willing to acknowledge their personal biases, prejudices, and ethnocentrism as blocks to therapeutic communication. Learning more about the cultures of your clients and accepting their uniqueness fosters therapeutic communication.

Common biases and prejudices in today's society include:

- A preference for Western medicine.
- Providers chosen according to gender.
- Prejudice related to a person's sexual preference.

- Discrimination based on race or religion.

- Hostile attitudes toward individuals with different value systems.

- A belief that people who cannot afford health care should receive less care than someone who can pay for full services.

Stereotyping

Self-Awareness

Stereotyping is to believe that all people or things with a particular characteristic are the same. Stereotyping says that all individuals of a particular culture are exactly alike. This philosophy is not true, even though individuals may share many cultural characteristics. It is important to recognize how personal perceptions may distort interactions with other cultures. Saying such things as "Mexicans always," "black people never," "all Italians belong to the Mafia," or any comments that stereotype a group of people can be very serious, and indicates a need for self-examination.

Health Care Rituals

Health care rituals are standardized procedures or protocols followed during a client visit. Some rituals are necessary from a medical point of view and others are not. For example, when children visit a dentist, parents may be asked to wait in the reception area during the examination. While this may be protocol, it may not be well received by individuals or clients from cultures who expect and feel more comfortable with the entire family coming along. Health care professionals must consider the rationale for such protocols and make exceptions when appropriate. The child coming for a first-time visit may need the security of the parent or caregiver during the examination. The parent or caregiver will be more comfortable staying behind at the next visit, knowing the child is familiar with what is going to happen and having seen professionals interacting with the child.

Language

Non-English-speaking clients may require the use of an interpreter for effective communication. In selecting an interpreter, the dialect of the client must be considered. For example, Chinese dialects may include Mandarin, Cantonese, or Shanghainese. Each dialect is unique, with its own cultural nuances. Dialect, as well as **regionalism**, may also be encountered with English-speaking clients. Clients from Scotland, while speaking English, can have a brogue that is almost incomprehensible to Americans.

Another language barrier compounding communication problems is the unique meanings given to different words based on the experience, culture, and ethnicity of the client. For example, people in some locations may use the term "tennis shoes" whereas other areas may refer to the same shoe as "sneakers." African Americans sometimes use a language termed **African American Vernacular English (AAVE)**, known colloquially as *Ebonics*. The example in the opening case study, referring to the doctor as "bad," is an example of AAVE, and actually is a complimentary statement meaning "very good."

When communicating with culturally diverse populations, people who speak English as a second language (ESL), also referred to as English speakers of other languages (ESOL), will be encountered. Many ESL clients have not learned to *think* in English and must first translate the English words into their native language, process the thought, and then translate it back into English before responding. This will require the health care professional to speak more slowly, use simple terms, and to realize there may be a delay in receiving a response from the client.

It is also important to remember that the process of communicating differs among cultures: It involves *how* the message is said, *when* it is said, and *why* it is said. Understanding various cultures and their values, beliefs, and communication styles will greatly enhance effective multicultural communication.

When working with non-English-speaking clients or clients with limited English-speaking skills, it is vital that these limitations not be perceived as limited intelligence. In their own language, clients may be able to fluently discuss their health care needs. It is only the language limitation that gets in the way of understanding. Also, just because a client does not understand English is not a reason to speak louder. It is better to use a normal tone of voice and speak a little slower, while enunciating each word clearly and using simpler vocabulary words. Allow clients extra time to process what is said and to form a response.

Perceptions and Expectations

Perceptions are insights or intuitions; it is the ability to see, hear, or become aware of something through the senses. Perception takes sensory data and personalizes it into images of reality. Synonyms for perception might be recognition, awareness, consciousness, and realization. Study Figure 2-2 closely. Two entirely different images emerge, depending on whether the eye is focused on the image or the white background. Can you see the old woman and the young girl? In health care, perceptions must be verified and validated in order to prevent misunderstandings.

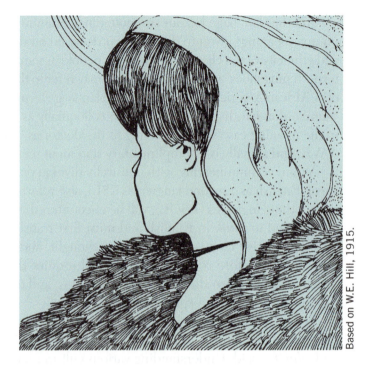

Based on W.E. Hill, 1915.

FIGURE 2-2   Young Girl and Old Woman Optical Illusion.

Cultural

Expectations are the events we anticipate based on experience or communication. ⊕ We usually expect clients to use the same communication style and language as we do. In some Asian countries, it is not polite to have eye contact with someone who is older or considered superior, yet in Western culture, it is common and even expected to have eye contact. Similarly, in Arab countries it is considered an insult to show the sole of your shoe facing another person. When expectations do not match with reality, confusion and misinterpretation frequently occur and therapeutic communication is stifled.

DEFINING CULTURAL EXPECTATIONS

A good place to start in defining the cultural characteristics of a client is to utilize some of the cultural domains identified in the Purnell model for cultural competence, and to formulate questions to define each domain. Five of the 12 domains in the Purnell model are appropriate to multicultural therapeutic communication. Table 2-1 defines the domains and the points that describe each domain.

TABLE 2-1   **Cultural Domains and Their Content**

Domain	Content
Communication	Language spoken
	Context
	Volume or tone of speech
	Body language
	Sensitivity to touch
	Comfort zone
	Eye contact
Family Roles in Health Care	Head of household and gender roles
	Principal caregiver
	Role of extended family
Health Care Practices	Focus of health care
	Traditional practices
	Folk medicine
	Magic/religious/traditional beliefs
	Pain
	Self-medication/prevention
	Acceptance of medical procedures
	Expectations
Health Care Practitioners	Perception of practitioners
	Gender of practitioners
	Folk practitioners
Spirituality	Spirituality and health
	Prayer
	Meaning of life
	Religion/religious practices
	Religious taboos

Each of the domains can be identified by observation, by research, or by asking questions related to each of the elements making up a domain. It might be possible to have the client complete a questionnaire to find out many of the answers. This would also evaluate the client's ability to follow instructions and to communicate in writing.

CROSS-CULTURAL COMMUNICATION

Communication between cultures speaking the same basic language can be difficult as a result of context and body language. They may have a major influence on communication between medical personnel and clients.

Two styles of communication context are defined: low- and high-context. **Low-context communication** utilizes few environmental or cultural idioms to convey an idea or concept, but relies mainly on explicit and highly detailed language. **High-context communication** involves great reliance on body language, reference to objects in the environment, and culturally relevant phraseology to convey an idea. The stereotype of Native American communication shown in old American Westerns exaggerates high-context communication. The preceding sentence is also an example of high-context communication as it requires cultural knowledge of old American Western movies. High-context communication assumes that the speaker and the listener both have knowledge regarding the subject.

No communication style is superior to another; the important thing to remember is that both the speaker and the listener should be cognizant of the style being used. The high-context style involves painting a word picture based on common experiences shared between the speaker and the listener. If both individuals do not share the same experiences, the word picture is not focused and miscommunication results. Conversely, the low-context style requires that the vocabulary of the listener be at least equal to the spoken vocabulary of the speaker.

People from cultures utilizing different context styles often develop an incorrect impression of one another. Low-context communication is direct and "in your face," whereas high-context communication is indirect and seems to take forever to reach a conclusion. The high-context speaker is often thought of as being less educated or mentally slow, whereas the low-context speaker is often thought of as being rude because of the directness of his or her speech. Neither of these perceptions is necessarily correct. Table 2-2 presents the characteristics common to high- and low-context cultures.

TABLE 2-2   **Characteristics Common to High- and Low-Context Cultures**

Category	High-Context	Low-Context
Relationship	Trust is slowly established	Aloof, shallow relationship
	Trust is developed before transacting business	Goal oriented
	Interpersonal relationships are important	Rank related to accomplishments
	May be offended by legal contracts and lack of trust	Social structure is broad
	Rank or status is based on group identity	
	Outsiders are not readily accepted	
	Closed circle of associates	
Communication	Indirect or implicit verbal picture message	Direct message is conveyed by words
	Nonverbal elements are important	Straightforward explicit meaning to communication
	Disagreement is personalized	Little attention to nonverbal communication
	Consensus is very important	Authority trumps consensus
Spatial Orientation	Space is shared	Privacy is important
		Person has private space requirement
Time Focus	Schedule is not important	Schedule is all important
	Cultural change is slow	Action oriented
	Time repeats or is circular	Change is accommodated
	Past oriented	Time is important
		Present or future oriented
Learning Mode	Group orientation/problem solving	Individual orientation/problem solving
	Deductive reasoning	Inductive reasoning, factual
	Intuition	Focus on detail, task centered
	Teamwork is preferred	Learning by explanation from others
	Learning by observation and practice	Specific to general
	General to specific	Efficiency and speed are valued
	Excellence and completeness are valued	

(*continues*)

TABLE 2-2   **Characteristics Common to High- and Low-Context Cultures (*continued*)**

Category	High-Context	Low-Context
High/Low Situations	Family gatherings, gatherings of close friends, tightly knit groups, medical staff, twins	Sporting events, cocktail parties, public meetings
High/Low Context Places/Cultures	Asia, South America, Africa, Middle East, Native Americans/Pacific Islanders, French speakers	United States, Canada, Northern Europe, Scandinavia, Australia, New Zealand, Israel

Caregiving Structure

Legal

The caregiving structure in a given culture can impact the relationship between medical personnel and clients when it comes to treatment and care. Most adult Caucasians from a Western culture are individualistic and take responsibility for their medical requirements and care. Other cultures, however, do not share this philosophy. This can result in problems with privacy considerations and client adherence to prescribed treatment. In cultures where the principal caregivers are relatives or extended family, the client may find it difficult to understand why these caregivers cannot have access to information about their medical condition and test results without written consent. In some cultures it is quite common for caregivers to accompany a client into the examination room. Special efforts must be taken to ensure compliance with Health Insurance Portability and Accountability Act of 1996 (HIPAA) requirements while accommodating for the client's wishes.

Time Focus

The cultural background, as well as the socioeconomic environment of individuals and cultures, determines their focus regarding time. We have an inherent built-in tendency toward a specific time focus that shapes how we think and act. Time focus can be oriented toward future, present, or past. A review of Maslow's Hierarchy of Needs, found in Appendix A, will be helpful before continuing this section.

Individuals having a *future time focus* are usually confident that their basic needs of food and shelter will be met, and are willing to sacrifice immediate gratification for better returns in the future. Future-oriented individuals are very time conscious and plan out their day and lives in considerable detail. They are usually prompt for appointments and expect the same of others.

Individuals with a *present time focus* are less assured that their needs will be satisfied. It is difficult to develop future plans when the basic items in the Hierarchy of Needs have not been met. It is interesting to note that in cultures where basic needs are provided in abundance, there is also the tendency to have a present time focus. This is possibly due to seeing no reason to improve things in the future. Even after economic status improves, tradition and culture can dictate a present orientation in many groups for generations to come.

Artificial limits placed on economic advancement, by a class system or racial or ethnic discrimination, may also cause people to have a present time focus, since improved future status is not an option open to them. Religion can also influence people to adopt a present time focus. Many religions encourage reliance on a spiritual being to provide for daily needs, and believers are encouraged to live day to day. Other religions consider time to be circular, like an endless ring, making time irrelevant. Children in almost all cultures are present focused. Present-oriented people, regardless of the reason for the orientation, do not look on time as being as important as do future-oriented people, and tend to be careless about promptness. It should be clarified that this is not usually out of any disrespect for the other person.

Past time focus is associated with culture and longstanding tradition. Past-oriented people revere traditions and usually honor elders, both living and dead. Asian and Native American cultures frequently exhibit some past orientation. Because past-oriented cultures see time as continuous and repeating, they are not as time conscious as future-oriented people. Because of their respect for elders, however, they usually try to please; hence, promptness is a characteristic if they respect the other person or if the person is considered educated.

We can force our time focus to change. Present *needs* must be met, however, before a present-focused person can transition into a future-focused person. The goal for time focus should be a mixture of future, present, and past. The past focus should be on positive experiences and not reliving negative experiences.

THE CULTURE OF FOLK MEDICINE

There is an increasing trend toward integrative medicine, which includes complementary therapies, being embraced by both Western-style and non-traditional practitioners. In some areas of the United States, **folk medicine** or old home cures may be used for all illnesses except serious ones. Folk medicine employs home remedy medications without a scientific understanding of the processes involved, and usually has been handed down from earlier times. For example, the wormwood plant has been used to treat fevers in China for 2,000 years. Recently a compound found in the wormwood plant has been used in a new antimalarial drug. The Hispanic culture uses chili peppers to treat pain. Today pharmaceutical companies utilize capsaicin as a topical cream for arthritis pain. Appalachian-influenced cultures advocate a tablespoon of black strap molasses in their coffee for extra iron. Wooly salve, a candle-like stick that is melted and dropped on an area that contains a splinter, thorn, or bee stinger was used to draw the foreign substance out.

Many folk medicines are beneficial, or at least do not cause harmful effects; others, however, are considered dangerous. An example of a dangerous drug is *azarcón* or *greta*. It is used to treat stomach ailments in Guatemala. The drug contains lead and is known to cause seizures, coma, and even death. Another example is *kava kava*, an herb used by Pacific Islanders to make an anxiety-relieving tea. Drinking a concentrated form of this tea poisons the liver.

Folk healers practice in their homes or in a religious setting. There are many names given to these healers. Examples include grannies and herbalists, whose learning has been primarily passed down from generation to generation. Spiritual healers, known as *shamans*, describe receiving their gift during profound religious experiences. They are more likely to use prayer, laying-on of hands, and holy oil or water with supernatural powers to heal. Supernatural healers may be referred to as sorcerers, voodooists, or root doctors.

Clients who take folk medicine most likely will not readily share this information with their health care professionals. Therefore, it is important to listen carefully when taking the client history, observe the client carefully without being judgmental, and ask questions about the illness and any remedies or treatments they may have tried. Clients involved in folk medicine may wear charms, amulets, or copper or silver bracelets believed to protect or warn of illness and may provide cues for health care professionals in treatment protocols.

EFFECTS OF CULTURES ON HEALTH CARE

Cultural

⊕ Case Study: Multiculturalism

You call your new client, Wangui, and escort her to the exam room. As you walk with her you introduce yourself and can't help but notice her attire as it is quite different from other clients. Her hair is in tight braids and is pulled back at the nape of her neck. She is wearing a colorful turban-like head dress and a brightly colored top and long skirt. Once in the exam room, you ask the reason for her visit today. Speaking with a slight accent that sounds a little British, she tells you she has had headaches for weeks now. They seem to be getting more intense. You notice that she is wearing a beautifully carved stone around her neck and wonder if this could be a talisman.

Culture has a greater effect on the attitudes relating to medical treatment and therapeutic communication than race and physical characteristics. Culture determines conscious and unconscious beliefs, learned behaviors, and likes and dislikes in clothing and food that develop from life experiences. Paradigms, the unconscious part of our culture, result in behaviors or choices that may mystify both client and medical personnel. For example, a client's unwillingness to be treated by a female provider may result from the paradigm that all providers are male. Understanding cultural paradigms may be the greatest challenge encountered during therapeutic communication. In trying to define a culture, individual beliefs and values must not be forgotten. Unless we understand individual aspects of cultures, we will not be able to facilitate effective therapeutic communication. The generalizations portrayed in the following descriptions should not be construed as cultural stereotypes. They are only a starting point in defining a client's culture.

Caucasian, Western Culture

People of Caucasian, Western culture have a high acceptance of Western medicine, relying on pharmaceutical products and surgical procedures to treat illness and disease. They lean toward preventative medicine and, generally, are not afraid to question medical opinion. They often take the time to complete extensive research regarding their condition. This enables the client and provider to discuss the problem and various methods of treatment in depth. This group is characterized by self-reliance, with the client or a member of the immediate family serving as caregiver.

African American, Western Culture

People of African American, Western culture are similar to the Caucasian, Western Culture; however, there are still many cultural characteristics unique to this group. The greatest difference is in how they focus on time. This group more likely has a present time focus that can result in placing less importance on punctuality, and a lesser disposition toward preventative medicine. The extended family is the predominant caregiver for African Americans; this can present a problem with the HIPAA regulation for privacy unless steps are taken to obtain authorization for release of information from the client. People of African American culture are sometimes distrustful of medical personnel of other cultures. This presents a barrier to successful therapeutic communication when it occurs.

African or Caribbean Culture

People of African or Caribbean culture accept Western medicine, but often exhibit a predisposition toward home remedies combined with cures based in spiritualism. The primary caregiver is a relative or a member of the "extended family," which may include people having tribal affiliation. Extended family includes all people the client looks to for trust and support. These cultures are basically present time focused and do not lean toward preventative medicine.

Stop and Consider 2.2

Cultural

⊕ Reread "Case Study: Multiculturalism", and respond to the following questions.

1. What questions might you ask in order to learn more about Wangui's culture?

2. What might you ask Wangui about her headaches?

Asian Culture

People of Asian cultures include many different subcultures (Asian, Indian, Chinese, Filipino, Japanese, Korean, Thai, Laotian, and Vietnamese). However, they each have enough similar cultural characteristics to permit treating them as a group. Medical personnel involved in treating primarily one or two of these subcultures may find it beneficial to study their individual cultural characteristics in greater detail.

This group, in general, accepts Western medicine; however, it can be strongly influenced by natural or folk medicine. Confucian principles of mind control over the body, maintaining a balance between natural forces, and eating foods designated "hot or cold" to treat illnesses are often embraced. This culture, along with people in surprising numbers from Western cultures, exhibit strong feelings regarding "saving face" or anything they perceive makes them feel inferior or ignorant. They will go out of their way to avoid insulting anyone. People of Asian cultures are usually present or past oriented, and display promptness as a symbol of respect. They will frequently smile and agree with a statement by nodding their head to avoid being disrespectful by challenging or questioning the speaker, or to appear not to understand. People of Asian cultures consider mental illness as shameful and deny anything they think suggests a mental condition. While the family is primarily patriarchal, the mother, and sometimes the grandmother, are the primary caregivers. This cultural group is quite private, speaks quietly, and does not believe in touching, especially the head, as it is considered sacred by some and the carrier of the soul.

Native American/Pacific Islander Cultures

Native American and Pacific Islanders accept Western medicine. However, spirit beliefs, "Mother Nature," or natural control of events in their lives are frequent influences. There is a great reliance on folk medicine and spiritual cures for illness. They do not readily speak of illness, as many believe that to do so may cause the problem to occur. This belief is significant to the medical professional, in that it results in an unwillingness to discuss a current illness or to practice preventative medicine. This culture is present focused and uses high-context communication, using few words. Eye contact is considered disrespectful; they are quiet and frequently show little emotion. Medical professionals need to exercise care to avoid confusing these cultural traits with disinterest or defiant noncompliance. The primary caregiver is the extended family and may include members of their tribe.

Hispanic and Latino Cultures

People of Hispanic and Latino cultures are present focused, and accept Western medicine. However, some have an equally strong belief that the Christian God has control of their lives and that illness may be the result of sins against God. This can result in a fatalistic approach to treatment, or the idea that penance or other works on their part are required to cure an illness. As a result, the medical professional must be very careful in communicating treatment protocols and the importance of compliance. Showing respect by using direct eye contact is recommended to obtain cooperation in treatment. The extended family is involved in health care, with the mother or grandmother serving as principal caregiver.

Stop and Consider 2.3

Cultural

⊕ A Malaysian mother brings her 12-month-old infant in for his annual physical examination.

1. How might the health care professional explain the necessity of procedures and their relationship to growth and development patterns?

2. How will you demonstrate respect for this culture in your therapeutic communication?

Religion-Based Cultures

Religion can have as great an impact on communication in a medical setting as culture. People with a strong belief that their God will take care of all healing and who expect miraculous cures may be unwilling to allow themselves or their children to be treated by health care professionals. Those who believe in spiritualistic rituals and charms, or who rely on folk medicine prescribed by lay healers, may not follow the type of care prescribed in Western medicine. Still others will not allow the provider to do his or her job in diagnosing and treating an illness because the examination may violate a religious prohibition considered more important than life itself. Medical personnel involved with any of these groups must seek to identify the barriers to effective medical care and try to work within their framework to gain the confidence and respect of the client, so that therapeutic communication and treatment can result.

The key to overcoming barriers resulting from the religious convictions of clients is to understand their religious background. The health care professional will want to have a nonjudgmental attitude regarding religious symbols and books that bring peace and comfort to clients in times of stress are essential (Figure 2-3). Being sensitive to the prohibitions and folk cures inherent in that religion or belief and discussing with the client how they can be incorporated into treatment can overcome these barriers.

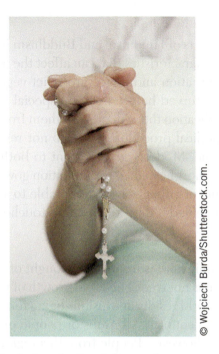

FIGURE 2-3   Be sensitive to the client's religious preferences.

Judaism

Practitioners of Judaism worship on the Sabbath (from sunset Friday to sunset Saturday) versus Sunday for most Christians. They consider the Sabbath as a day of rest, and Orthodox Jews limit doing even such simple things as turning on a light switch or appliance. Scheduling medical tests or procedures on the Sabbath should first be discussed with the client.

Normal hospital routine is usually acceptable to people practicing Judaism, with the exception of dietary restrictions revolving around eating pork and food preparation techniques. Kosher food is available in most modern Western hospitals, but when it is not, vegetarian food and dairy products are frequently acceptable. During Passover, leaven is to be avoided. Judaism allows most tests and procedures as long as they preserve human life. Abortion is strictly prohibited. Mutilation of the body is forbidden, and this can cause some problem when an autopsy is required. Autopsy is allowed only when mandated by civil authorities. Judaism does not have special rituals involving dying clients, except that they should be attended by a chaplain or rabbi at the time of death.

Hinduism and Buddhism

Practitioners of Hinduism and Buddhism have similar religiously influenced cultural characteristics that can affect the medical practitioner. Both believe in reincarnation and hence are strict vegetarians. Buddhists may require meals be served before noon on special feast days. Buddhists may refuse pain medication that will prevent them from being mentally alert and aware. Most medical procedures that do not result in the destruction of life are acceptable. Modesty is important to both Hindus and Buddhists; consequently, short hospital or examination gowns will often be refused. Medical personnel of either sex are acceptable to all except priests. Priests are considered defiled if they touch or are touched by a woman.

Islam

The Islamic faith is frequently thought of as Middle Eastern or Arab; however, that is not true. The rapid growth of people embracing Islam throughout the world results in Muslims being found in almost every cultural ethnic group and country. All Arabs or people of Middle Eastern culture are not Muslims, however. People from this region are Muslim, Christian, or Jewish, with the majority being Muslim. According to a 2013 Pew Research survey, a significant portion of the population is prejudiced against Muslims. They further believe that any person who claims Islam as their religion has been radicalized. This is an incorrect generalization.

Embracing the Islamic faith drastically changes the believer's inherent culture. The resulting modified culture differs significantly from their original culture. The male head of the household makes most decisions, even for a female client, and the immediate family is the primary caregiver. In some instances, it may be required that the male family members be told medical information prior to telling the client. Muslims are modest in dress, precluding a display of body parts; hospital or examination gowns are highly objectionable and many will refuse to wear them. Strict followers of Islam may not allow a female to be touched or examined by a male provider, and a woman who has never been married cannot have a pelvic examination due to concern that it may affect virginity. When a woman is examined, another person of the same sex must be present. Male Muslim clients may object to a female being in charge of their nursing care or as their provider.

Dietary requirements are part of Islamic-influenced culture. Nonpork or even a vegetarian diet may be followed, and alcohol is prohibited even as a base for medications. Daily prayers are part of the life of a strict Muslim, and not being allowed to follow this requirement can cause discomfort. Ritual washing is a part of the preparation for prayer, as is washing private areas after using the toilet. The client's physical condition and availability of facilities will dictate the feasibility of compliance, but if at all possible the staff should comply with such requests to achieve the best recuperation and recovery from illness.

Miscellaneous cultural traits or taboo subjects exist in the Islamic faith that can interfere with medical treatment. Touching by people of the opposite sex is frowned upon, and shaking hands upon greeting is frequently not done even between men. Mental illness is not acceptable, and since birth defects are considered a test of their faith, they are frequently ignored and not discussed. Muslim clients are generally fatalistic and do not readily accept a terminal disease because they believe that God controls all things. Hospice care is not usually acceptable to Muslims. These restrictions are only part of an extensive list of taboo subjects, and represent those that would be most likely to offend a person practicing Islam.

Christian Science

Christian Scientists believe that all illness and suffering is illusory. They believe that illness results from a mistaken view of reality, indicating a need for spiritual renewal. While not denying that infection is of bacterial origin and accepting modern diagnostics, they believe that all forms of disease are symptomatic of underlying conditions requiring spiritual healing through prayer. They do not believe that drugs have a real power and their effect is solely the result of false human consciousness and as such the effect is only temporary.

While individual members are free to seek modern medical treatment, they are encouraged to seek help from Christian Science practitioners and nurses. The practitioners have limited medical knowledge and are trained for a ministry of healing through consultation with the ill person, discussion of Christian Science principles, and prayer. The nurses complement the practitioners, offering nonmedical physical care conducive to spiritual healing. A practitioner will not treat a Christian Science member while they are being treated using modern Western medicine. Christian Scientists, however, may seek hospital or midwife assistance for childbirth. They comply with requirements for legally required vaccines, requirements for quarantine, reporting infectious diseases, and having mandatory physical examinations. They will seek medical aid for fractures and dental emergencies. They will also use pain medication for severe pain until they can apply Christian Science treatments.

Table 2-3 summarizes the information regarding cultural and religious effects on health care presented in this section.

TABLE 2-3   Generalization of Cultural/Religious Effects on Health Care

Culture or Religion	Medical Care Background	Caregiving Structure	Communication Traits	Time Focus*
Caucasian, Western culture	**Western medicine,** rely on prescription medications, practice preventative medicine, may rely on folk medicine	**Individual,** immediate family, close friends	**Low-context,** direct eye contact expected, not adverse to therapeutic touching, may challenge medical opinions, basic English, speaks loudly	**Future**
African American, Western culture	**Western medicine,** rely on prescription medications, practice preventative medicine, may rely on folk medicine	**Extended family,** relatives, close friends, neighbors, church family	**Low-context,** direct eye contact expected, not adverse to therapeutic touching, may challenge medical opinions and can distrust medical personnel, basic English sometimes mixed with AAVE	**Present**/future
African or Caribbean culture	**Mixture** of Western medicine combined with spiritualism	**Extended family,** relatives, close friends, neighbors, church family, tribal affiliation	**Low-context,** eye contact expected, highly emotional, basic English strongly mixed with local dialect	**Present**
Asian culture (Asian, Indian, Chinese, Filipino, Japanese, Korean, Thai, Laotian, Vietnamese)	**Mixture** of Western medicine combined with Confucian principals (i.e., mind control of the body and maintaining a balance between natural forces and energy in the body), eating foods designated as having hot and cold properties to cure illness is common, mental illness is considered shameful and is denied	**Immediate family,** opinions of family and particularly elders are important	**High-context,** indirect, avoid eye contact, show little emotion, avoid therapeutic touching, youth speak basic English, elders may speak little English, may agree with what is said even when they do not understand in order to avoid conflict or to avoid losing face, speak softly	**Present**/past
Native American/ Pacific Islander cultures	**Mixture** of Western and folk medicine combined with importance of a balance between the forces of nature	**Extended family,** relatives, close friends, neighbors, tribal affiliation	**High-context,** avoid eye contact, speak softly and slowly, basic English mixed with tribal dialects	**Present**

	Health/Medicine beliefs	Family	Communication	Time focus*
Hispanic and Latino cultures	**Mixture** of Western and folk medicine combined with a strong belief in intervention by God, eating foods designated as having hot and cold properties to cure illness is common	**Extended family,** relatives, church family, collective community	**High-context,** be respectful and make direct eye contact, speak softly, some basic English, most speak Spanish	**Present**/past
Judaism	**Western medicine,** religion does not allow eating pork and requires kosher food	Culturally dependent	Culturally dependent	**Future**/present
Hinduism/ Buddhism	**Western Medicine,** religions do not allow eating meat, modest regarding their body	Culturally dependent	Culturally dependent	**Future**/present
Islam	**Mixture** of Western and folk medicine combined with a strong belief in intervention by Allah; match gender of caregiver and client, woman may not be permitted to be examined by male medical professional, mental illness denied, do not ingest alcohol, believe complete rest is proper for all illnesses, do not eat pork	**Immediate family,** opinions of family and particularly male head of house hold are important	**High-context,** touching between men and women is prohibited for strict believers, do not discuss sexual dysfunction, females do not make direct eye contact, will not discuss many taboo subjects (mental illness, birth defects, contraception, hospice), those from Middle East speak loudly to indicate the importance of what they are saying	**Future**/present
Christian Science	Most are unfamiliar with Western medicine, preferring to rely on prayer and spiritual intervention; accept clinical diagnosis, but attribute the causation to an underlying spiritual condition, do not believe healed by prayer; do not believe in drug therapy and may reject vaccination; each has freedom to seek modern medical treatment	**Immediate family** and the use of Christian Science practitioners and nurses committed to a ministry of healing, but none have medical training or knowledge	Christian Scientists could have any cultural background and hence communicate in the context of that culture; because of their lack of medical knowledge, the provider should clearly explain any procedures	**Present**/future

*stating that the bold term represents the predominant focus

OVERCOMING LANGUAGE AND AUDITORY BARRIERS

Legal

The Americans with Disabilities Act (ADA) requires that health care facilities—both public and private, large and small—provide effective communication alternatives to people with language and hearing loss or speech impairment. The provider can choose the communication method or device as long as it results in effective communication. The expense for this accommodation must be charged against the overhead of the clinic and may not be billed to the client.

A language deficiency can be overcome by using an interpreter, employing a human translator, using a telephone or service translator, or using online translation systems with software applications such as *Google Translate, Speak and Translate, FaceTime,* or *Skype.* These applications can translate in real time with text or with voice recognition software. Current technology has the capability to translate some 100 languages. The main disadvantage of voice systems is that they require speaking slowly and have difficulty translating technical terminology. When a person-to-person interpreter has been considered to be the translation mode used in the clinic, a resource list of interpreters should be compiled. The Registry of Interpreters for the Deaf, Inc. is an excellent resource (*www.rid.org*). Your local city or state registry of interpreters may also be useful. It is also important to document the mode of preferred communication within the client's medical record.

Using a Medical Interpreter

A medical interpreter facilitates communication between non-English-speaking clients and health care professionals. These individuals are trained professionals proficient in the knowledge and skills of cultural and medical language, and are employed in health care settings. They respect the values of diverse cultures and variations within health care systems and are knowledgeable about both. They are able to overcome existing language barriers, so that everyone understands each other clearly and mutual trust is fostered. They also have a working knowledge of possible community services for clients who may need support other than health care; examples include housing, food, clothing, and childcare.

The use of an interpreter is especially helpful when consent forms are required, assessment questions are asked, and specific instructions are given to the client. Interviews of this nature require cultural sensitivity and an awareness of any legal and ethical implications. Using interpreters can increase the quality of care provided to clients. They aid the provider in acquiring a complete and accurate medical history to enable diagnosis and accurate documentation of health care issues. When clients understand what is required for treatment, they are usually more compliant, willing to sign the necessary consent forms, and follow treatment protocols.

Guidelines for using an interpreter include the following:

- Brief the interpreter. Discuss the reason for their presence and review the types of questions that may be asked during the interview and any goals to be achieved.

- Introduce the client and interpreter and allow them some time to establish a rapport before the interview begins.

- Assure the client that confidentiality will be maintained and that nothing will be shared without the client's written permission to do so.

- During the interview, position yourself so that you can see both the interpreter and the client, but maintain appropriate eye contact and direct questions to the client. Observe the client's nonverbal communication.

- Keep it short. Avoid long or complicated sentences during the interview. Focus on one subject at a time (i.e., "Do you have pain?" not "Do you have pain, tiredness, or loss of appetite?").

- Do not interrupt a conversation between the client and interpreter.

- Allow the interpreter, as well as the client, time to think. Do not be impatient.

- Be aware that the client may understand some English.

- Be sensitive to cultural diversity regarding age, gender, and socio-economic status between the client and the interpreter. For example, selecting an interpreter who is of the same gender and similar age as the client may be helpful in some cultures. When working with Asian cultures, it may be wiser to choose an interpreter who is older than the client and is viewed by the client as someone to be respected.

- Allow time with the interpreter after the interview has been completed. This permits the interpreter to share anything that could not be shared in the client's presence, or to offer insight relating to impressions regarding nonverbal cues or culture preferences.

- Use the same interpreter for any follow-up visits.

The Therapeutic Response

When interacting with clients of different cultures, the following basic communication techniques will be helpful.

- Develop knowledge of the cultures of the clients in your care and assess their values, cultural health care practices, and expectations.
- Know as much as possible about the culture's communication style. Listen to the words clients use to express concerns and incorporate these words into your verbal response.
- Determine the degree of cultural assimilation. Does the client dress in traditional clothes? A client who is still embedded in the original culture may not have much contact with the predominant cultural group and may present a greater challenge in the client relationship.
- Unobtrusively assess how recently the client has immigrated to the United States. Try to understand the environment in their parent country (i.e., war, dictatorial government, and immigration by choice or due to terrorism). Sensitivity to any client who may be undocumented and recognition that some of these situations may result in distrust and lead to lack of openness are important.
- Create an atmosphere that is comfortable and respects the clients' personal space as well as their cultural, lifestyle, and religious preferences.
- Approach the clients slowly and respectfully. Do not touch or offer to shake hands with the clients until you have assessed their cultural background.
- Recognize and respect the culture's nonverbal mannerisms and gestures. Ask the clients to repeat in their own words any instructions back to you to ensure understanding.
- If language is a significant barrier, consider using an interpreter.
- During the client interview, in addition to asking symptoms, ask clients what they think caused the illness and what treatment they think should be used to treat the illness. The clients might also be asked how the illness was treated in the past.
- Use reflecting questions or statements to validate the feelings and concerns of the clients. This encourages clients to share more completely.

- Allow sufficient time, and try not to rush the client.

- Does the client follow traditional dietary customs that could interfere with the prescribed course of treatment? Folk medicine coupled with modern drugs may cause unwanted or unknown interactions. On the other hand, traditional dietary habits of native peoples are often healthier than American eating habits because there is little use of processed foods or overuse of animal fats. In fact, modifying the client's native dietary pattern may make a disease such as diabetes easier to manage than if the client ate a typical American diet.

- Do not belittle folk medicine and unless it is contraindicated, consider allowing its continuation in order to develop the trust and respect of the client.

- Consider prescribing common folk treatments to achieve the medical results desired. An example would be prescribing healthful, cultural beverages such as a specific herbal tea to maintain hydration instead of simply prescribing water.

- Do not jump to conclusions based on your own culture and belief systems.

SUMMARY

Learning more about cultural diversity is a very enriching experience. Each culture is unique; each is good; one is not better than another; one may be more familiar to us, but that does not make it better. It is important to practice techniques that build and foster multicultural therapeutic communication. This involves learning about the beliefs and values of different cultures and religions and recognizing any barriers, including biases or prejudices that may impact multicultural therapeutic communication. Using an interpreter who is able to interpret the client's language and specific cultural nuances, as well as health care culture and terminology, aids the medical team in providing the best health care. When possible, consider allowing any procedures or alternative treatments that are comforting to the client and that are not detrimental to the treatment regimen being prescribed.

EXERCISES

Exercise 1

Using the following questions, assess your own cultural background, recognizing that cultural values are principles or standards that members of a cultural group share in common. Each background will have both shared values and individualized values.

1. Identify your culture.

2. List three cultural values that your culture possesses.

3. List three cultural values that are important to you as an individual.

4. Discuss how these personal values directly relate to your heritage or culture's attitudes, beliefs, and behaviors.

5. Discuss how your cultural values have influenced the way in which others perceive and react to you.

Exercise 2

First, define the meanings of *bias* and *prejudice*. Using the columns provided, list cultures, religions, and sexual orientations, and any biases and prejudices you recognize in yourself when communicating with these diverse groups.

Culture, Religion, Sexual Orientation	Biases	Prejudices

What steps might you initiate to decrease these biases and prejudices?

Exercise 3

Visit a market in an ethnic neighborhood.

1. Describe the market.

2. Were you familiar with any of the foods or items sold in the market?

3. Describe the shoppers and the sales personnel in the market. How did they interact and communicate?

4. What was your comfort level while in the market?

5. Did you find or observe any biases toward *you*?

Visualize the market as a health care facility, with you as the client and the sales personnel representing health care professionals.

6. What could the market sales personnel have done to make you feel more comfortable?

7. From the marketplace experience, develop a written plan of what you could do in a health care setting to make the experience more comfortable for a person of another culture.

REVIEW QUESTIONS

Multiple Choice

1. What are three important factors to consider when developing multicultural therapeutic communication?

    a. Learning about the beliefs and values of different cultures, practicing using barriers to cultural communication, and participating in discussions with multicultural individuals

    b. Determining your own cultural beliefs, practicing using barriers to cultural communication, and participating in discussions with multicultural individuals

    c. Learning about the beliefs and values of different cultures, recognizing any barriers to cultural communication, and practicing techniques that build and foster multicultural communication

    d. Determining your own cultural beliefs, practicing techniques that build and foster multicultural communication, and practicing using barriers to cultural communication

2. What is the meaning of ethnocentrism?

   a. A slant toward a particular belief.

   b. The belief that one's own culture and traditions are better than those of others.

   c. An opinion or judgment that is formed before all the facts are known.

   d. Usually a preconceived and unfavorable concept.

3. Juan arrives at the clinic 40 minutes late for his follow-up visit. With a great deal of gestures and mannerisms, he explains that the fog and rain delayed him. Which communication context style has Juan demonstrated?

   a. High-context communication   **c.** Low-context communication

   b. Nonverbal communication   **d.** Verbal communication

4. Mary Beth's sense of belonging and trust has been shaken since her second divorce. She is most often late for appointments and is very impulsive. What is Mary Beth's time focus?

   a. Past time focus   **c.** Western time focus

   b. Eastern time focus   **d.** Present time focus

5. Dr. Yamaki approaches different cultures slowly and respectfully. He engages in conversation that will help him assess the clients' cultural health care practices and values. Which type of communication does this represent?

   a. Nonverbal communication   **c.** Low-context communication

   b. Therapeutic communication   **d.** High-context communication

6. An opinion or judgment formed before all the facts are known is termed:

   a. prejudice   **c.** racism

   b. ethnocentrism   **d.** bias

7. What is the speech or manners representative of a specific geographical location termed?

   a. Regionalism   **c.** AAVE

   b. Dialect   **d.** Rituals

8. Can you describe the progression through Maslow's Hierarchy of Needs?

   a. Physiological, love and belonging, safety, esteem, and self-actualization

   b. Love and belonging, safety, esteem, physiological, self-actualization

   c. Esteem, love and belonging, safety, physiological, self-actualization

   d. Physiological, safety, love and belonging, esteem, self-actualization

9. What percentage of the meaning and intent of communication is by spoken words?

   a. 83%   c. 7%

   b. 10%   d. 20%

10. Which of the following is not accurate of the ideal interpreter?

   a. Interprets the client's language

   b. Interprets an equivalent meaning of the client's response

   c. Interprets the client's specific cultural nuances

   d. Should not be selected with age, gender, or socioeconomic status considered

FOR FURTHER CONSIDERATION

1. How can you, as a health care professional, recognize the uniqueness of each culture, including your own, and incorporate this uniqueness into therapeutic communication?

2. When language is a communication barrier, how might the health care facility take steps to ensure that therapeutic communication is possible?

3. Preconceived negative biases or prejudices about clients of different cultures hamper therapeutic relationships. How might the health care professional assess personal negative biases or prejudices?

4. Using the Internet and your favorite search engine, investigate a culture that you are not familiar with. Print out pages related to this culture and discuss similarities and differences between various cultures with a classmate.

5. Now that you have finished studying this chapter, are there changes you will make personally in your therapeutic communications with multicultural clients?

CASE STUDIES

Case Study 1

A health care professional attempted to explain infant care techniques to Iranian parents. Since the mother was not feeling well, the health care professional began explaining everything to the husband. He refused to listen, stating that in his country, men did not get involved in childcare.

1. Using information from this chapter and research through the Internet, investigate cultural values and beliefs of Middle Eastern families.

2. What therapeutic communication techniques would be appropriate in this situation?

Case Study 2

Mr. Suzuki, a Japanese man in his 70s, recently experienced a stroke that resulted in right-side weakness. He spent several weeks in a rehabilitation center relearning self-care activities and tasks involved in daily living. His therapist spent a great deal of time with Mr. Suzuki and his family, explaining through practical instruction how these skills could be accomplished. Mr. Suzuki and his wife sat passively through the instructions. During the therapy sessions with staff members, Mr. Suzuki was compliant and made good progress in relearning self-care activities, and was able to walk using a walker. When Mr. Suzuki was back in his room, he expected his wife to do everything for him, even self-care activities that he did for himself during therapy sessions.

1. Use the Internet to learn more about Japanese values and beliefs regarding health care and family.

2. Identify the cultural characteristics that may be potential problems in Mr. Suzuki's rehabilitation.

REFERENCES AND RESOURCES

Doing a cultural assessment. (n.d.). *EuroMed Info*. Retrieved from www .euromedinfo.eu/doing-a-cultural-assessment.html.

Gates, G. J., & Newport, F. (2012). Special report: 3.4% of U.S. adults identify as LGBT. *Gallup*. Retrieved from www.gallup.com/ poll/158066/special-report-adults-identify-lgbt.aspx.

How culture influences health beliefs. (n.d.). *EuroMed Info*. Retrieved from www.euromedinfo.eu/how-culture-influences-health-beliefs.html/.

Humes, K. R., Jones, N. A., & Ramirez, R. R. (2011, March). Overview of race and Hispanic origin: 2010. *2010 Census Briefs*. Washington, DC: U.S. Census Bureau. Retrieved from www.census.gov/prod/cen2010/briefs/c2010br-02.pdf.

Lindh, W. Q., Pooler, M. S., Tamparo, C. D., & Dahl, B. M. (2014). *Comprehensive medical assisting: administrative and clinical competencies* (5th ed.). Albany, NY: Thomson Delmar Learning.

Luckmann, J. (2000). *Transcultural communication in health care*. Albany, NY: Thomson Delmar Learning.

Novickas, R. (2014, January/February). Helping Hands: Reach out to deaf and hearing-impaired patients. *CMA Today*.

Pew Research Center. (2013). 45% say Muslim Americans face "a lot" of discrimination: After Boston, little change in views of Islam and violence. Retrieved from www.people-press.org/files/legacy-pdf/5-7-13%20Islam%20Release.pdf.

Purnell, L. D. (2014). *Culturally competent health care*. Philadelphia: F.A. Davis.

Somashekhar, S. (2014, July 15). Health survey gives government its first large-scale data on gay, bisexual population. *Washington Post*. Retrieved from www.washingtonpost.com/national/health-science/health-survey-gives-government-its-first-large-scale-data-on-gay-bisexual-population/2014/07/14/2db9f4b0-092f-11e4-bbf1-cc51275e7f8f_story.html.

Tamparo, C. D. (2016). *Diseases of the human body* (6th ed.). Philadelphia: F. A. Davis.

Ward, B. W., Dahlhamer, J. M., Galinsky, A. M., & Joestl, S. S. (2014). Sexual orientation and health among U.S. adults: National Health Interview Survey, 2013. *National Health Statistics Reports, 77*. Retrieved from www.cdc.gov/nchs/data/nhsr/nhsr077.pdf.

Chapter 3
Therapeutic Communication in Complementary Medicine

CHAPTER OBJECTIVES

After completing this chapter, the learner should be able to:

- Define key terms as presented in the glossary.

- Recall current statistics for the use of complementary and alternative medicine (CAM) in the United States.

- List at least five common characteristics of individuals who use CAM.

- Compare traditional or allopathic medicine to alternative medicine.

- Contrast traditional or allopathic medicine to complementary medicine.

- Diagram the educational requirements and licensure status of both the alternative medicine practitioners and the traditional practitioners identified in this chapter.

- List alternative medical therapies identified in this text with a brief description of their practices.

- Provide examples of the negative and the positive components of both the alternative and the traditional therapies for medical care.

- Examine the rationale and hesitation of both traditional and nontraditional practitioners to embrace integrative medicine.

Opening Case Study

Alicia is 64 years old. She has taken an early retirement from teaching. She is an outdoors person and enjoys hiking, climbing mountains, and snow skiing. A year ago, she hiked to the bottom of the Grand Canyon with a group of women similar in age. She spends her time between two homes—one in the mountains, the other by the seashore. She is active in a number of community organizations and in her church. She is a skilled gardener. Alicia also has severe osteoarthritis and sciatic pain from lumbar spinal stenosis.

Alicia's orthopedic specialist has said that surgery is a possibility, but Alicia refuses. She fears "going under the knife," and has chosen to manage her pain in a different manner. She has prescription medication to manage her most serious pain, and has gone the route of injected corticosteroid drugs on two separate occasions.

Alicia believes that she must stay active. Except on the days when pain is nearly unbearable, she attends a spinning class at a local gym and follows up with an hour of yoga. She also does "hot yoga" when the pain is really rough. She is consistent in doing the exercises given to her by both the orthopedic specialist and a physical therapist.

Stop and Consider 3.1

1. What do you think of Alicia's health management plan?

2. Do you believe that Alicia may do damage to her body with such a serious exercise regimen? Justify your response.

INTRODUCTION

Alternative health care is embraced by a large number of individuals in the United States. Interestingly enough, it is also likely paid for personally rather than by insurance. In 2010, nearly $34 billion was spent by individuals for alternative health care. The National Center for Complementary and Integrate Health (NCCIH; established in 1998 by the U.S. Congress) and the National Center for Health Statistics (NCHS; part of the Centers for Disease Control and Prevention) indicate that over 38% of adults and 12% of children in the United States are using some form of complementary and alternative medicine. The 2012 National Health Interview Survey, conducted by the NCHS, revealed a number of interesting facts regarding the use of complementary and alternative medicine (CAM):

- Recognizing the role of psychological distress on general health leads to increased acceptance of a **biopsychosocial** model of health care.
- Women and middle-aged people are more likely to embrace CAM.
- CAM use increases with education and income, perhaps due to the knowledge of alternative therapies.
- The chronically ill use CAM five times more than the average population.
- Participants of CAM generally desire a greater control over one's health and dissatisfaction with traditional **allopathic medicine**.
- Many clients do not share their participation in CAM with their primary care provider (PCP).
- Insurers gain when clients opt for CAM for many of the noncovered services. This occurs because when insurance does not pay for noncovered services, they pay out less dollars and create more profit.
- Many traditional or allopathic practitioners will embrace certain types of CAM in order to increase their cash flow as well as respond to clients' demands.

It is also evident that clients turn to CAM not only for the control they believe they gain, but because they perceive that their PCP often appears too busy (often because some insurance carriers reward providers based on the number of clients seen) and more interested in providing a medication's "quick fix" for an ailment than to spend time on getting to the root of any problems presented. These clients seek a provider who gives more time and attention to their needs, creating the perfect rationale and opportunity for therapeutic communications in complementary medicine.

HEALTH CARE MODALITIES DEFINED

Western, traditional, or allopathic medicine is generally the most familiar health care modality to Americans. **Western medicine** is based on the premise that disease results from bacterial and viral attack on the body. Diseases are diagnosed by observing the clients' symptoms and from scientific tests. Treatments consist of pharmaceutical products and surgical procedures, as appropriate. Mental state is recognized as contributing to wellness, but receives less consideration in most treatment regimes.

The PCP who is a medical doctor (MD), osteopath (DO), or chiropractor (DC) generally fits into this category. All three are licensed to practice in all 50 states. Primarily, the modality practiced by these providers is based on the development of microscopy, bacterial cultures, radiography, and medications. Osteopathy and chiropractic also add manipulation of bones and joints, especially of the spinal column, to their treatments. Education of the MD and the DO is very similar in training and length of time. The DC completes 4–5 years of specialized study in an accredited chiropractic college.

Alternative, complementary, or integrative medicine is quite varied in education, training, and licensure requirements. Complementary medicine by its definition "complements" traditional therapy or works in tandem with traditional medicine. Alternative medicine does not always "complement" traditional medicine; in fact, it may work against traditional medicine. Refer to Table 3-1 for a listing of both major traditional and nontraditional health care practitioners.

The doctor of *naturopathy* (ND) receives 2 years of science courses and 2 years of clinical work based on "natural" and nontoxic medicine, nutritional supplements, and physical modifications in breathing and posture. NDs currently are licensed in 16 states and the District of Columbia. *Homeopathy* practitioners believe healing takes place when miniscule amounts of certain substances are able to leave an imprint in the body, stimulate the immune system, and help facilitate a cure. They are licensed only in Arizona, Connecticut, and Nevada.

Traditional Chinese medicine (TCM) is an ancient modality referring to the five elements of fire, earth, metal, water, and wood. The common goal is to strengthen the body's immune system and increase its capacity for maintaining health. TCM practices likely include Asian, Pacific Islander, American Indian, and Tibetan cultures. TCM believes the key to health is *Qi* (pronounced "chee"), the "life energy" that flows through the body along meridians in order to create harmony and balance. Yin (the feminine element) and yang (the masculine element) are important concepts of TCM.

TABLE 3-1   Education and Training for Traditional and Nontraditional Health Care Practitioners

Practitioner	Practice	Education	Licensure
Medical doctor (MD)	Allopathic or traditional	BS + medical school and 3- to 7-year residency	All 50 states
Osteopath (DO)	Allopathic with spine manipulation	Same requirements as MD	All 50 states
Chiropractor (DC)	Spine manipulation; pharmaceuticals and surgery *not* included	Undergraduate coursework + 4–5 years specialty study	All 50 states
Naturopathic doctor (ND)	Nontraditional	BS + 2 years science; 2 years clinical	Currently licensed in 16 states
Homeopathic doctor	Nontraditional	3–4 years in homeopathic program	Licensed in AZ, CT, and NV
TCM practitioner	Ancient modality of yin/yang	BS + 3–4 years of specialty training; Masters in Oriental Medicine available	Often licensed as acupuncturists
Acupuncture	Ancient practice of needle piercing along 365 points and 12 meridians of the body	BS + 2 years specialty training	Varies by state
Ayurveda	Ancient practice of balance and harmony	1,500–2,500 hours meets National Ayurvedic Medical Association requirements	Not licensed in any state
Mind/body therapists	Psychoneuroimmunology, hypnotherapy, imagery, etc.	Individual states set training standards	Individual states determine licensure requirements

TCM may use herbal medicines, **moxibustion**, **Qigong**, **acupressure** or **acupuncture**, and **cupping** in treatment. Many states license acupuncturists (Figure 3-1). To learn more about Acupuncture and Oriental Medicine education and state requirements, visit www.nccaom.org.

The *Ayurvedic* practice of medicine comes from India where it is delivered as a primary healing tradition, and is as ancient as TCM. The belief is that if there is a balance and harmony of body, mind, and spirit, then health and the absence of disease will follow. Diet, sleep habits, and the use of herbs are used to address health issues. Also included are aromatherapy, meditation, and yoga. For additional information, visit https://nccih. nih.gov and search for "Ayurveda." No states currently license Ayurvedic practitioners.

Mind/body therapies are suggested by many of the above practitioners. It is believed that the mind and the body are equally significant medically. Biofeedback, **psychoneuroimmunology**, hypnotherapy, imagery and visualization, and journaling exercises are possible therapies employed. Of note, music, dance, tai chi, and art therapy are also often used in mind/body therapy. Recently, animals have been introduced and used in therapy in hospitals, skilled nursing facilities, and assisted-living communities. There is evidence that when a person pets a dog or a cat who returns that loving affection, blood pressure goes down and the heartbeat slows. Some nursing facilities have a resident dog or cat. Research links the immune system to

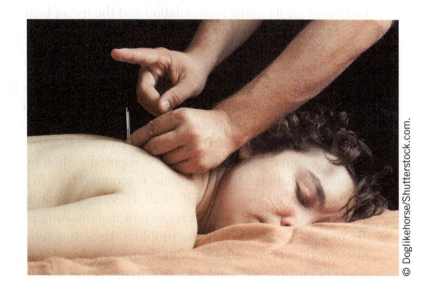

© Doglikehorse/Shutterstock.com.

FIGURE 3-1   A TCM practitioner performs acupuncture on a client's shoulder.

the brain to show how illness, mood, stress, and thought play a role in one's general health. All these therapies fit into the category of enhancing the immune system and making an individual less susceptible to disease.

Massage and therapeutic touch are closely related to the practice of osteopathy and chiropractic treatments. There are a number of different forms of massage, but basically it is the manipulation of soft body tissues to enhance health and well-being. Massage is often used to relieve pain, reduce stress, release adhesions or scar tissue, and provide greater range of motion and flexibility. *Therapeutic touch* is based on the premise that all human beings have a system of energy layers in constant interaction with the environment, others, and themselves. Illness occurs when this energy field is out of balance. Therapeutic touch therapists place their hands near and around the client's body, allowing their energy field to interact with the client's energy field. This process is designed to clear or rebalance the energy field and promote the body's own natural healing ability.

WORDS OF CAUTION

In reading this material, you probably have identified practices you personally embrace or believe are valid. Keep in mind, however, that the only modalities based on scientific knowledge and research are classified in the Western medicine grouping. However, even chiropractic should be embraced for its spinal manipulation and the use of heat, ultrasound, massage, and electric muscle stimulation to manage some muscle and bone issues, rather than the belief that **subluxations** cause ill health that spinal adjustments can cure.

Naturopathy can become dangerous with excessive fasting, repeated enemas, and colonic washings. The use of unregulated herbs often infused with impurities and harmful substances can interact with conventional drugs and become dangerous. Homeopathy also has limits. Not all conditions respond to micro doses of substances, especially when surgical intervention or an immediate relief of symptoms is required (i.e., in an asthma attack).

TCM has its limits as well. If all TCM treatment was as beneficial as artemisinin, the world's most important malaria drug isolated in TCM by Tu Youyou, there would be no problem. Unfortunately, many of the mixtures used in TCM contain toxins, heavy metals, added steroids, and even traces of endangered animal tissues. Acupuncture has shown effectiveness in managing pain, but is not recommended for anyone who bleeds easily or is taking blood thinners. Acupuncture may give a person increased energy and mental clarity for a brief time. For anyone with a pacemaker, electrical impulses to the needles can cause interference to the pacemaker.

The three body energies or **doshas** of Ayurveda can be helpful to any medical practitioner wanting to determine what and how a person's energy might contribute to ill health. To maintain proper balance in a person's doshas, herbal medicines, dietary changes, yoga, massage, and breathing exercises may be recommended, but are not known to cure many common ailments and diseases. Also, the herbal medicines can have the same problem described earlier with impurities and harmful substances.

Massage has many positive components, but should be avoided in anyone with fractures, severe osteoporosis, thrombocytopenia, deep vein thrombosis, burns or open wounds, and bleeding disorders. Therapeutic touch can be used with any traditional medical treatment, but is inappropriate for serious or life-threatening situations or to replace proven treatments for treating illness.

Yoga has long been touted as a beneficial exercise to promote flexibility and posture. When there is no physiological reason not to participate, it can be very helpful. Hot yoga, however, presents issues for consideration. Not all individuals are comfortable in a super-heated environment (perhaps to over 100 degrees Fahrenheit) while exercising. The heavy sweating can result in dehydration, decreased blood pressure, increased heart rate, and a feeling of weakness, nausea, and dizziness. Heat exhaustion can occur. Clients are advised not to participate in a hot yoga class if the instructor does not permit anyone to leave the room when these symptoms are experienced. In a super-heated environment, increase in blood flow makes it seem as though you are more flexible than is really the case. Remember that the more the ligaments are stretched, the greater the risk of tearing one.

The Therapeutic Response

It is important to remember that anyone who embraces alternative or complementary therapies probably has personal reasons for doing so. Recall, too, the numbers of individuals entering into these therapies on a daily basis. The best approach is to interview clients carefully and with sensitivity regarding their participation. No alternative or complementary therapy should be explored without the approval and understanding of the PCP. Many of the modalities described here can complement traditional therapy,

(continues)

The Therapeutic Response   (*Continued*)

and often provide less-invasive treatment plans, but they can also work against the same therapy when caution is not exercised.

Be reminded, too, that a traditional practitioner or physician may not be all that excited about a client's choice of an alternative therapy because the very term "alternative" means that the therapy is used to "replace" the more traditional therapy. Likewise, there will be practitioners in the nontraditional route who will see no advantage to cooperating with traditional physicians. Therefore, bringing complementary and traditional or allopathic medicine together in an integrative approach to client-centered care is really the goal. All the facets of communication identified in previous chapters will further facilitate this communication process.

Stop and Consider 3.2

Reflect again upon the case study in the beginning of this chapter.

1. Would you suggest any cautions to Alicia about her regimen? Explain your response.

2. What forms of nontraditional medicine have you embraced? Were they alternative or complementary? Did you tell your PCP of your choices?

SUMMARY

Alternative and/or complementary therapies are growing in popularity for treating diseases in today's world. The increasing population of immigrants coming to the United States only heightens this fact as they may come with non-Western approaches to medicine that often challenge the traditional practitioner. That challenge, however, can enhance and complement the overall approach to treatment when cooperation and communication is open and honest.

EXERCISES

Exercise 1

Explore the Internet to determine if there are any warnings or dangers to your choices of complementary or alternative medical care. Will you make any changes?

Exercise 2

Select just one of the alternative or complementary therapies identified in this chapter that particularly interests you. With the use of the Internet, make a list of both the positive and negative aspects of this therapy.

REVIEW QUESTIONS

Multiple Choice

1. What is the percentage of adults and children using CAM in the United States?

    a. 38% children and 12% adults

    b. 48% adults and 15% children

    c. 38% adults and 12% children

    d. 78% adults and 10% children

2. What is the practice of a PCP with similar education and training as an MD who also is able to manipulate the bones and joints?

    a. Chiropractic   **c.** TCM

    b. Osteopathy   **d.** Homeopathy

3. Simon has tried everything for his back pain and is fearful of the narcotics he often has to take to get through his work on a construction site. What nontraditional therapy might be suggested?

    a. Surgery   **c.** Imagery

    b. Homeopathy   **d.** Acupuncture

4. What therapy attempts to strengthen the immune system and increase its capacity for maintaining health emphasizing the five elements?

    a. Allopathic medicine   **c.** Naturopathic medicine

    b. TCM   **d.** Mind/body therapy

5. What therapy requires 2 years of science courses and 2 years of clinical work?

    a. Ayurveda   **c.** Naturopathy

    b. Chiropractic   **d.** Hypnotherapy

6. What are the common characteristics of individuals who embrace CAM?

   a. They have lower than average income and are mostly male.

   b. They have no health insurance and are usually female.

   c. They are likely educated, middle-aged women with a high income.

   d. They are younger males seeking control over their health insurance.

7. What do insurers of health care gain when clients opt for noncovered CAM services?

   a. Insurers do not have to pay claims for these services.

   b. Insurers have fewer claims to process.

   c. CAM services provide a threat to providers that insurers are trying to control and manage.

   d. Insurers do not have to check the licenses of CAM practitioners.

8. What reason(s) might a traditional practitioner have for including the practice of a nontraditional provider in his or her own clinic?

   a. There is another person to provide "after-hour" services.

   b. The traditional practitioner may be moving toward integrated medicine practices.

   c. The facility's reputation will be enhanced.

   d. Profits will be doubled.

9. What are the dangers in using herbal medicine?

   a. They are hard to purchase in the local pharmacy.

   b. The Food and Drug Administration says herbal medicines are illegal.

   c. The purity of herbal medicines makes them very expensive to use.

   d. Harmful substances in herbals may interact negatively with traditional medicine.

10. What definition would you use to describe integrative medicine?

   a. Integrative medicine is used instead of allopathic medicine.

   b. Integrative medicine combines the best of Western and complementary medicine.

   c. Integrative medicine is the same as alternative medicine.

   d. Integrative medicine combines alternative and allopathic medicine.

FOR FURTHER CONSIDERATION

1. What key factors will you consider when addressing a client who is or has embraced nontraditional therapy for their medical use?

2. What therapies suggested in the text have the benefit of boosting the immune system?

CASE STUDIES

Case Study 1

Harl is 87 years old. He winters in Southern California. He needs to have major dental work and is quite shocked at the prices quoted to him by two dentists in the California area. He talks with others in his retirement community who encourage him to seek a dentist across the border in Mexico.

1. What do you think of this plan?

2. Do a little research to determine how common it is to seek medical attention in another country. Is the only reason because of the decreased cost? If Harl has problems after his dental work is completed in Mexico and he returns to the United States, what might occur?

Case Study 2

You are the only daughter to your mom who lives more than 1,500 miles away. You are beside yourself with excitement to tell her about the news—she will become a grandmother in a few months. You go on to tell her of your wishes to use the services of a **doula** when it is time for the baby to be born. Your Mom, however, is not the least bit excited about your choice of a doula—that is, after you tell her what a doula is.

1. What does a doula do? Why might this practice appeal to an expectant mother?

2. What can you do to calm some of your Mom's anxiety?

3. What is the attitude of obstetricians to doulas?

REFERENCES AND RESOURCES

American Cancer Society. (2013). Naturopathic medicine. Retrieved from www.cancer.org/treatment/treatmentsandsideeffects/complementaryandalternativemedicine/mindbodyandspirit/naturopathic-medicine.

Clarke, T. C., Black, L. I., Stussman, B. J., Barnes, P. M., & Nahin, R. L. (2015). Trends in the use of complementary health approaches among adults: United States, 2002–2012. *National Health Statistics Reports*, 79. Retrieved from www.cdc.gov/nchs/data/nhsr/nhsr079.pdf.

Hall, H. (2013). Chiropractor's abuse: An insider's lament. Retrieved from www.sciencebasedmedicine.org/chiropractic-abuse-an-insiders-lament-2/.

Journal of Alternative and Complementary Medicine ISSN: 1075-5535. Online ISSN: 1557-7708. Current Volume: 21 (2014).

Kupferschmidt, K. (2012). Dangers of Chinese medicine brought to light by DNA studies. Retrieved from http://news.sciencemag.org/asia/2012/04/dangers-chinese-medicine-brought-light-dna-studies.

Lallaniaa, M. (2015). Ayurveda: Facts about Ayurvedic medicine. *Live Science*. Retrieved from www.livescience.com/42153-ayurveda.html.

Larsen, A. (n.d.). Hot yoga: The dangers and myths you need to know. *Breaking Muscle*. Retrieved from http://breakingmuscle.com/yoga/hot-yoga-the-dangers-and-myths-you-need-to-know.

Lindh, W. Q., Pooler, M., Tamparo, C. D., Dahl, B., & Morris, J. (2014). *Administrative medical assisting* (5th ed.). Clifton Park, NY: Cengage Learning.

Tamparo, C. D. (2016). *Diseases of the human body* (6th ed.). Philadelphia: F.A. Davis.

Treating cancer: Integrative medicine. Retrieved from www.drweil.com/drw/u/ART03060/Treating-Cancer-With-Integrative-Medicine.html.

Ullman, D. (n.d.). The limitations and risks of homeopathic medicine. Retrieved from www.homeopathic.com/Articles/Introduction_to_Homeopathy/The_Limitations_and_Risks_of_Homeopathic_Med.html.

Chapter 4
The Helping Interview

CHAPTER OBJECTIVES

After completing this chapter, the learner should be able to:

- Define key terms as presented in the glossary.

- Identify the purpose of the helping interview.

- Illustrate by example the three primary components of the helping interview.

- Contrast the feelings experienced by the individual giving help and the individual needing help.

- Assess the importance of a minimum of 10 preparations to be made by the health care professional before the interview takes place.

- Illustrate by example the following attributes and their use in the helping interview: risk/trust, warmth/caring, genuineness, sympathy/empathy, and sincerity.

- Provide examples of the following responding skills and their use: sharing observations, acknowledging feelings, clarifying and validating, and reflecting and paraphrasing.

- Discuss the levels of need and relate them to the helping interview.

- Differentiate how closed questions, open questions, and indirect statements encourage or discourage the therapeutic exchange.

- Describe how the following concepts block therapeutic communication: reassuring clichés/stereotypical comments;

giving advice/approval; requesting/requiring an explanation; belittling, defending, and changing the subject/shifting.

- Demonstrate the steps involved in an appropriate closure of a helping interview.

Opening Case Study

James Alonzo is on his way to the clinic of his primary care provider (PCP). He has no desire to do this. His wife made him come for a physical exam. It has been 5 years since his last one. He rarely sees a doctor. James had to take a couple of hours off work in the middle of a really busy project to keep his appointment. He steps into the clinic, goes up to the front desk, and gives his name. The receptionist asks for his insurance card and tells him to be seated. He wonders how long he will have to wait as he picks up a magazine. He says to himself, "The atmosphere in this place is about like the drive-up window for fast food."

After 20 minutes, a young woman comes to the doorway and calls out his name. He follows her down a hallway. She stops in front of the scale and asks him to step up. She jots the weight in his chart and takes him into the examination room. The conversation continues.

"So, I see you have come for a physical exam today."

"Yeah. My wife made me come, even made the appointment."

"Are you having any symptoms today? Are you taking any medications?"

"I take an aspirin occasionally, and antacids."

"How often do you take the antacids?"

"Oh, I keep them in my pocket, maybe once a day or so."

James kind of wants to talk about having difficulty emptying his bladder, but he is not about to tell this woman, especially when she looks as young as his high school–age daughter.

"I am going to take your blood pressure now. Please remove your shirt." James removes his shirt and puts it on his lap. When the assistant is finished, she tells James to take off all his clothes and put on a gown and Dr. Plano will be in shortly. James removes his clothes, but doesn't know what to do with his underwear, and wonders if he should leave his socks on. He waits another 10 minutes before Dr. Plano comes in.

"Good afternoon, James. What brings you in?"

"My wife says it is past time for me to have a physical."

(continues)

Opening Case Study (Continued)

"I see. It has been quite a while since you were in. You're 58 now, right? It appears your weight is up about 15 pounds and I see your blood pressure is somewhat elevated. We better address the antacids you're taking, too. Any particular problems you want to share with me?"

"Well, I kind of want to ask you about a problem I have when I pee. I can't seem to get it all out, and I have to go quite often. It is kind of embarrassing when I am standing in a public restroom at the urinal and everyone is done before I am."

"You might have an enlarged prostate. I'll know better after I examine you." As the doctor starts to listen to James's chest sounds, James begins to sweat. He is thinking, "Oh no! Prostate! If he has to do anything about that, I won't be any good at sex anymore."

Stop and Consider 4.1

1. How did the opening case study encourage communication? Explain.

2. In the discussion with James, what will the doctor focus on?

3. Will all of James's concerns be addressed?

INTRODUCTION

Seeking care in any type of health care facility is usually not the most favorite activity of any individual. It is likely viewed as a "necessary evil," something that must be done but is not pleasantly anticipated. Making the encounter between health care professional and client both helpful and therapeutic is a challenge. The techniques in this chapter will help to facilitate therapeutic communications between health care professionals and clients.

CHANGES IN TODAY'S HEALTH CARE CLIMATE

A large number of clients seeking care in today's health care climate come with far more information than ever before experienced in medicine. Consumers are bombarded daily by advertisements touting the claims of the latest medicines that are sure to cure the worst of ills and informing them of any and all possible side effects. Consumers already taking the prescribed medicine can become alarmed by the warnings given in the media; others, fearing they suffer from the described malady, are anxious to request the medication from their providers.

Many consumers are likely to conduct a fair amount of independent research via the Internet prior to seeking medical advice or accepting their provider's diagnosis or treatment plan. A second opinion is quite accessible via the Internet, and needs no recommendation from a doctor or insurance approval. PCPs, however, are concerned about the accuracy and validity of some information found on the Internet. Clients seeking medical information via the Internet do not always realize that such information is not specific to their particular case and does not take into account the same personal information their PCP has about them. While the vastness of the Internet may not provide the best information at all times, many consumers find it more accessible, friendlier, and less threatening than their provider's clinic and staff. Some sites on the Internet assist clients in making medical choices.

Consumers also may find their continuity of care interrupted by their employer's choices of health care plans, which can force a change in providers. For many, having the same PCP for a decade or more is increasingly uncommon. It becomes progressively more difficult to ensure that clients' complete health care records are in the hands of their current provider, even with the use of electronic medical records (EMRs). An issue with EMRs is that the many and varied software programs for EMRs rarely are able to communicate with each other. This means that an EMR created in one clinic may not be easily accessed by another clinic or hospital with different software. This problem creates a possible legal dilemma for providers, their clinics, the hospitals they serve, and for all clients with EMRs.

Legal

One of the most important aspects of the helping interview is empowering clients to become equal partners in their health care. The successful interview will help clients focus on their needs and encourage open and free "give-and-take" communication with their PCP. A closer look at the components of the helping interview and how to make it a successful encounter for both the client and the health care provider will help consumers receive the best possible medical care.

INTERVIEW COMPONENTS

A *helping interview* is a conversation between a health care professional and a person in need and is a common tool of communication in any health care setting. Three components of the helping interview are (1) the *orientation* of the professional and the client to each other, (2) the *identification* of the client's problem, and (3) the *resolution* of the client's problem. The helping interview is usually planned for a set time and place, with the health care professional in control. It is this control that often intimidates clients.

Control Factor

Control is a critical factor in the helping interview, but should not be abused. Even the use of the word *patient* implies a superior/inferior, higher/lower, more-knowledge/less-knowledge relationship. The helping interview clearly involves people in an unequal partnership. The provider has the power to provide or direct services required of the client or patient. Being in a state of need or helplessness is never empowering. Such a position requires trust in the one with the power and the belief that the one in power can be of assistance. Addressing the individual as a "client" rather than a "patient" returns some of that power to the person in need. Consider the following feelings likely to describe giving and needing help.

Giving Help Feels	Needing Help Feels
Important	Unimportant or inadequate
Useful	Useless or depressed
Powerful	Powerless
Gratified	Frightened or embarrassed
Happy	Sad or angry

Self-Assessment

It is more pleasant to give help than to need help. Health care professionals must be constantly aware of how their status affects persons seeking help. Clients should be empowered as much as possible by the experience in the helping interview, since empowered clients are likely to participate more fully in their care and return to health faster.

Orientation

There are some important preparations to be made by the health care professional even before the interview takes place. Personal appearance and the appearance of the medical facility or examination room are vital keys to getting the helping interview off to a good start (Figure 4-1).

Personal appearance and grooming must be professional and impeccable. The health care professional, always alert to the control of any

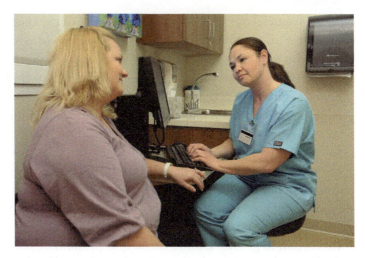

FIGURE 4-1   Give clients as much dignity and empowerment as possible.

disease-producing organisms, will remember that personal cleanliness helps reduce pathogens and inhibits their transmission.

Professional

The client expects a health care professional to look and dress the part. In fact, the client may have difficulty trusting someone who is too casual in appearance. A name tag that includes the title and credential is most helpful.

Consider the facility's surroundings. Is the reception area a pleasant environment where strangers can be seated comfortably with current magazines for their reading? Some facilities even offer large windows that allow sunshine and the viewing of a garden for relaxation. In the examination room, will the setting encourage an equal relationship? Are you seated near the client or with a desk between you? Is the examination room so small that the client must sit on the examination table? If possible, be seated facing the client and at the same level. The client should not, if at all possible, be disrobed during the orientation phase of the interview.

Greet your client in a pleasant manner and with a name when possible. Even in a busy clinic with a number of waiting clients in the reception area, it is not too difficult to identify the next client to be seen. Check the chart carefully to make certain it matches the client you are about to approach. Step close to the client to preserve confidentiality as you begin the helping interview. "Mr. Alonzo? Please come with me." Some clients bring another person with them, to accompany them during the actual examination. If this is the case, accommodations must be made for that individual. As you escort the client to the examination area, observe mobility and alertness.

Always match your pace to the client's, so he or she does not feel left behind, and offer any assistance that might be needed. Making "small talk" as you walk, you might comment: "I apologize for your wait; we got a little backed up today." Or, "Did you have trouble with traffic or finding parking?" If the client responds that there was difficulty finding parking, you might be able to respond, "I know it can be a problem, and sometimes I have difficulties, too. There are plans underway to create additional parking that will hopefully ease the situation." In this exchange, the client's issue is recognized and the self-disclosure of the health care professional fosters an atmosphere of trust. Do not ask, "How are you today?" Most do not feel well when they are seeking medical attention, so this cliché is not helpful.

Legal

Introduce yourself and give your title, as the client may not know it. Be certain to get the client's name and pronounce it correctly. In some facilities, clients are asked to give their date of birth and a photo ID. This is to ensure proper verification of the person being seen and the record in hand. Do not address the client informally unless the client requests that you do so. If the interview is conducted in an examination room, knock before entering.

Speak with a comfortable and appropriate tone and voice volume. Do not speak in a monotone. Make certain the client hears and understands you. If there is a language barrier or speech problem, get an expert to help you. Do not try to speak a language of which you really have only a little knowledge. Time is an important element; the health care professional must have time to hear the client. The helping interview is no place for misunderstanding.

Case Study: Professional Appearance

A recent newspaper features a student in a hair design school who went the "extra mile" when the school's instructor was approached for a special service. The request was for someone to come to the house where a young woman, age 26, was in the final stages of multiple sclerosis but wanted her hair cut. The woman, Amanda, who had been nearly helpless for 8 years, was currently receiving hospice care and living in the formal living room at her parents' small home. The instructor selected his best student, a man named Alan. Alan quickly replied he would be delighted to make the call, and asked another student to accompany him. Together they went to the home where they cut Amanda's hair, and added a manicure and a pedicure. They brought flowers to Amanda and were able to get her to laugh as they "toyed" with her hair to determine a style she might like. They refused payment and even swept the floor after the haircut when they finished. Amanda's parents were speechless.

Indeed, this scenario describes the very best of therapeutic communication and caring. What is not obvious unless you see the photos in the newspaper is that Alan is covered with tattoos—up and down his arms, on his hands, and on his face. He also wears earrings in his ears. While Amanda's parents were a little surprised at Alan's appearance, soon it made no difference at all.

Stop and Consider 4.2

1. Is there a difference in expectations between a health care professional and a hair designer regarding personal appearance? Discuss.

2. How can impressions make a difference in the communications between individuals?

3. What are the dress codes in your school? Are tattoos allowed? Explain the rationale.

Risk/Trust

As the interview gets underway, be aware that the conversation involves a fair amount of risk on the part of the client. Give all your attention to the client. Listen and observe. The health care professional needs to build an atmosphere of trust, making the risk easier. As the trust level increases, it is easier for the client to share feelings and attitudes about the problem. Trust has to be earned. Without it, the helping relationship will go no further than mere introductions. The health care professional is responsible for nurturing mutual trust.

Warmth and Caring

Warmth may be defined as an attitude expressing caring and concern. It is primarily communicated through facial expressions, such as a caring look or a smile, which cross all cultural differences. Often, the question "How can I help you today?" or a comment such as "I see you're here for a physical exam" is appropriate at this point. A calm, reassuring voice also expresses warmth and caring. Another expression of caring and warmth comes from the health care professional who gives full attention to the client and what is being said. Clients who sense that they are the most important person to the health care professional at that time are more likely to relax in a non-threatening atmosphere where they feel free to express concerns. *Caring* expresses a liking or regard for others, and communicates a watchfulness for cues that may indicate the problem and its possible solution.

Genuineness

Genuineness is being real and honest with others. The health care professional must be able to communicate honestly with others while being careful not to judge or condemn. Genuineness assures that there will be congruency between the verbal and nonverbal messages. Genuineness and acceptance are partners in the helping interview.

Sympathy and Empathy

To show *sympathy* is to respond to the emotional state of others and to acknowledge the feelings expressed by clients. Sympathy states, "I am available to you." *Empathy* is the ability to accept another's private world as if it were your own. It is fair and sensitive; it is an awareness of others' situations and what they are experiencing. It communicates identification with and understanding of another's situation. Empathy states, "I'm available to walk this road with you." Expressing sympathy and/or empathy encourages clients to express their concerns and helps them cope. The most therapeutic health care providers recognize that when they listen sympathetically to their clients, clients are better able to recognize their own completeness and strength.

Sincerity

Sincerity involves those attributes already identified, as well as creating an atmosphere that is free from hypocrisy. The sincere health care professional is forthright, candid, and truthful. Health care professionals must be sincere in their intentions and communications with others. Sincerity cannot be faked. If clients do not believe in your sincerity, they may "shut down."

IDENTIFICATION OF PROBLEM

Once the orientation phase has been completed and a trust level is established, it is time to turn attention to the problem or problems identified by the client. As well as remembering to listen with the "third ear" (i.e., being aware of what the client is *not* saying or picking up on hints as to the real message), there are a number of techniques that will ease the communication between clients and health care professionals. These techniques may be referred to as *responding skills*, and are identified in the next section.

Responding Skills

There are a number of skills for the health care professional to keep in mind during the helping interview.

Sharing Observations

Observations will focus on both the client's physical and emotional state. The statement "You seem a little anxious" conveys concern and interest in knowing more, and comes from the health care professional's observation of the client. The tone of voice, eye contact, and body position are all factors to be considered in observations. Statements such as "You are trembling" or "You seem to be in pain" are examples of shared observations (Figure 4-2). Such statements encourage the client to verbalize his or her feelings. Some professionals will ask a client to identify any pain he or she is feeling on a scale of 1–10, with 1 being mild and 10 being almost unbearable.

Acknowledging Feelings

Sharing observations is a way to acknowledge the client's feelings. This responding skill communicates to clients that their feelings are understood and accepted. It encourages verbalization by providing a safe, nonthreatening environment. An example of such an acknowledgment is "So does your wife

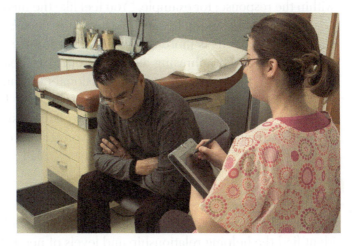

FIGURE 4-2   In observation of this client, what might he be experiencing?

have specific concerns that caused her to make the appointment?" or "I know not sleeping at night because of the cough is distressing and wears you out." Such acknowledgments make it easier for clients to reveal their symptoms.

Clarifying and Validating

Clarifying is used when the health care professional is not certain of the meaning of the message communicated. Such statements as "I'm not sure I understand what you mean" or "Do you mean . . .?" are examples of clarification. Words or nonverbal cues used during an exchange may hold different meanings for others, so clarifying is important. This is especially critical when languages or cultures are different or may be easily misunderstood. For example, shaking the head horizontally in most countries means "no." In India, shaking the head horizontally may mean "yes, no, or I don't know." When the thumb and forefinger form an "O" it means "everything is okay" in western European countries. In Japan, it means "now we may talk about money." In some Latin American countries, Eastern Europe, and Russia, it is an indecent sexual sign. For the message to be therapeutic, both parties must understand the same meaning, use the terms in the same manner, or understand the differences.

Cultural

Reflecting and Paraphrasing

Reflecting focuses on the emotional aspect of the client's expression. It involves listening to the verbal message as well as considering the nonverbal cues being sent. Facial expression and tone of voice will provide insight regarding the meaning of the message and its congruency. When using reflecting skills, "You feel" will often be used at the beginning of or within the response; for example, "You feel like the medicine is not helping."

Paraphrasing simply restates in the professional's own words what the client said. Its focus is more on the cognitive aspects of the message than on the feelings. Paraphrasing allows the client to hear what was just said and to verify the accuracy of the professional's listening ability. It is often helpful to tie together reflecting and paraphrasing. Using words such as "You feel . . . because . . ." connects the two skills easily; for example, "You feel the medicine is not helping because you still have the headaches."

LEVELS OF NEED

A number of years ago, Paul Welter, in his book *How to Help a Friend* (1990), identified the helping relationship and levels of need. To become an effective helper, it is necessary to recognize what level of need your client has.

TABLE 4-1   **Levels of Need**

Level and Definition	Characteristics of Person in Need	Effective Helping Response
Problem Has a solution.	Asks specific question; wants immediate advice or information.	Supply information or advice.
Predicament No easy solution.	Often feels trapped; is not helped by advice.	The helper gets involved; works for openness.
Crisis A very large predicament; short term.	Has a sense of urgency; may want help but is afraid to ask.	Expects you to help; bring client into present; accept emotions.
Panic A state of fear; sees only one way out.	Does not listen; mind is caught in dreadful future event; nonrational.	Move client from panic to "hold"; use touch, eye contact.
Shock A numbed or dazed condition.	Fails to take action; mind lapses for short time; unable to recall lapse.	Must act for this person. Stay with this person until back to normal.

Based on Welter, P. (1990). How to help a friend. Wheaton, IL: Tyndale House Publishing.

Although this chart was established for helping friends, it can be adapted to recognizing the needs of clients who come for help. See Table 4-1.

Appendix A (see p. 277) provides a section about psychologist Abraham Maslow, who developed criteria for determining a person's needs. He believed that individuals move back and forth from one need to another, depending on their circumstances. Clients seeking treatment for medical problems are likely to be experiencing both physiological and safety needs.

Recognizing that clients have different levels of need helps professionals to focus their attention correctly. Keeping in mind the attributes identified and the levels of need creates an atmosphere in which clients can ask questions that will assist them in fully identifying the problems they face.

QUESTIONING TECHNIQUES

Real skill is involved in knowing how to ask questions in a manner that helps the client express problems. These questions and answers are important to the identification and resolution of the problem. Also, they become the foundation for the client's medical record. There are three major types of questions that are useful during the helping interview, and each has its own appropriateness.

Closed Questions

Closed questions are useful in collecting information during the client history, and are most common at the beginning of the verbal exchange. They do not require the individual being asked the question to enlarge upon the answer. The questions usually begin with *do*, *is*, or *are*, and are answered with a simple *yes*, *no*, or a brief phrase. Examples of closed questions are as follows:

"Are you experiencing pain now?"

"Does it hurt when you raise your arm?"

"Can you feel the lump when you are lying down?"

Open-Ended Questions

Open-ended questions are most helpful for therapeutic communication, as they encourage clients to identify more of the problem. They do not put words into clients' mouths; rather, they allow them to express their own thoughts and feelings. Open-ended questions usually begin with *how*, *what*, or *could*. They are an invitation for clients to express more detail. Examples of open-ended questions are as follows:

"Could your new job be responsible for a change in your eating habits?"

"What foods seem to trigger the need for antacids?"

"What did the doctor tell you about this medication?"

Indirect Statements

Open-ended questions can be reworded so that they become indirect statements. Indirect statements call for a response from the client, but do not make the client feel like he or she is being questioned. They do, however, encourage verbalization and express interest in the client from the health care professional. Examples of indirect statements are as follows:

"I'd like to hear about your new therapy program."

"Tell me what worries you most about this problem and how it affects your daily life."

"Let's discuss what makes it so difficult for you to quit smoking."

During the helping interview, it is beneficial to stay away from the use of questions that begin with *why*. When questions begin with *why*, clients often become defensive or feel they are being accused. Questions beginning with *how* or *what* are much more effective. This and other roadblocks to communication are identified in the next section.

ROADBLOCKS TO COMMUNICATION

There are so many roadblocks to communication that one marvels at how any communication is effective. In therapeutic communication, preventing roadblocks is vital to a quality relationship with the client.

Some of the most common roadblocks to therapeutic communication are:

- Reassuring clichés
- Requiring explanations
- Defending
- Moralizing/lecturing
- Giving advice/approval
- Belittling/contradicting/criticizing
- Changing subject/shifting
- Shaming/threatening/ridiculing

Health care professionals must keep in mind that when clients seek care for some problem or ailment, they have delicate psychological and mental attitudes and must be handled with care to put them at ease. It also must be remembered that every communication is a transcultural one. Therefore, paying close attention to communication roadblocks is vital.

Reassuring Clichés

Reassuring **clichés** are often given automatically, and consist of patterned responses; trite expressions; or empty, meaningless phrases that express false assumptions about how a client feels. When the health care professional senses the client may be anxious or stressed, reassuring clichés may be expressed in an effort to reduce these feelings. However, the client will likely interpret clichés to mean the professional does not understand the problem or is not interested in becoming involved. These phrases also may be used by health care professionals to reduce their own personal anxieties. Examples of reassuring clichés are as follows:

"Everything will be all right."

"Keep your chin up. Hang in there."

"Just do it!"

Giving Advice/Approval

Self-Awareness

Giving advice may occur when health care professionals act from a subconscious desire to have all the answers, or feel the need to control the client's thoughts or actions. This usually occurs when the health care professional is doing more talking than listening. When clients are told what they should do, opinions and solutions are imposed on them. This advice-giving usually begins with "If I were you . . ." or "You should . . ." Recognition of the fact that these phrases are being used should trigger a warning signal to stop. No one can ever be in the exact circumstances or situations of another person. Remember, the goal is to sufficiently empower the client, who will then be able to recognize what advice might be needed. Even when the provider gives directions to clients, the phrase used should be "My recommendation is . . ."

Requiring Explanations

Asking clients to explain their reasons for feelings, behaviors, or thoughts requires them to analyze and explain these experiences. Questions that ask *why* are intimidating. Examples include "Why do you think you are feeling this way?" and "Why did you do that?" Often clients may not understand the reasons for the discomfort to begin with. They may understand the discomfort but not know how to describe it, or they may not have sufficient trust in the health care professional to risk sharing their feelings. During the helping interview, health care professionals should ask clients to describe their feelings rather than explain them. This approach is non-threatening and communicates to clients that their feelings are acceptable. It encourages clients to continue describing their situation.

Belittling/Contradicting/Criticizing

Expressions such as "There is no way you bled that much" or "You shouldn't feel that way" send a message to the client: "You are mistaken; your feelings are unimportant." When a client comes with a concern or a complaint, responding negatively will close the communication process immediately. The client feels what the client feels. Even if the professional knows that what is being described is impossible, clients are still the only ones who know their own body and feelings. Listen to and acknowledge the client's statements. Do not contradict.

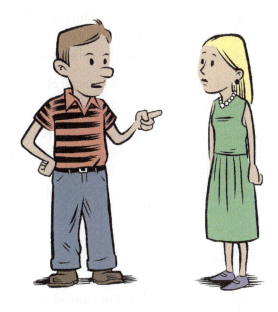

"YOU SHOULDN'T FEEL THAT WAY."

There is *never* a time in a therapeutic relationship when a client should be criticized. Even if a client does something that is foolish, harmful, and extremely unhealthy, criticism does not open the lines of communication for wise, safe, and healthy advice or information.

Defending

"There is no way the doctor will discharge you today." When the health care professional defends something or someone the client has criticized or contradicts a client's statement, it implies the client has no right to express his or her feelings, concerns, or impressions. This contradiction will block the therapeutic exchange and prevent further verbalization by the client. Communication has closed.

Changing the Subject/Shifting

When the health care professional changes the subject or shifts to new topics, the direction of the conversation will be controlled by the professional rather than allowing clients to discuss freely what they choose. Shifting the trust of the helping interview toward the health care professional's perceptions also blocks the exchange. Once the client has been blocked, he or she may discontinue future attempts to share feelings, concerns, or problems. An example of changing the subject or shifting is as follows:

Client: "I have decided not to have any more chemotherapy."

Professional: "Did your daughter visit this week?"

The professional might change the subject because he or she is uncomfortable with the topic or simply may want to gain information related to another specific subject. Care should be used in changing the subject or shifting to a new topic, to be certain it is appropriate to the present verbal exchange.

Moralizing/Lecturing

Health care professionals who easily criticize probably moralize also. Even if the client appears with a condition caused by a lifestyle that is totally contrary to society's standards of health, expressing judgment is unlikely to have a positive effect on the client. To moralize is to be unable to fully and completely accept the client's needs. In Elaine's situation, described in Chapter 1, her self-esteem was partly preserved by the refusal of her health care professionals to moralize over her decision. Health care professionals who work daily with persons who abuse substances must not moralize, but must be able to see the person that he or she was or who can be again.

Self-Awareness

Health care professionals, with all their knowledge and many years of experience, are apt to lecture. They might feel the lecture is quite appropriate to the situation, but even when the sharing of information is vital to the client's well-being, to lecture only makes the client feel defensive or of little value.

Shaming/Threatening/Ridiculing

To ridicule or shame a client will close communication immediately. Most often, this ridicule or shame is in the form of nonverbal rather than verbal communication. Health care professionals have been taught not to ridicule or shame, but these behaviors often show in actions rather than words. To laugh at a client's description of an ailment or misunderstanding of basic body functions is a common example of ridicule. To threaten a client with the consequences of some act only causes fear, submission, and resentment. It does nothing to encourage the client to change behavior. Clients are able to determine for themselves if their actions are damaging and what the consequences will be. Health care professionals who threaten are usually insecure or feel total responsibility for their clients. Neither characteristic is healthy.

RESOLUTION OF THE PROBLEM

As the helping interview nears completion, a couple of questions can be asked to make certain that clients have had the opportunity to express all their concerns. These questions might be "Is there anything else you would like to ask me today?" "Are there any other concerns that you have?" As the helping interview comes to a close, it is hoped that some resolution of the problem is also obvious. While many problems will require ongoing care, there should be some problem resolution in each helping interview. It is important for the health care professional to use the clearest and simplest language possible, since most clients have little or no knowledge of medical terminology. It is important to remember that if the receiver has not understood the message as it was sent, no communication has taken place.

Most clients seek an explanation for their problem, and want to know how the resolution of the problem is going to affect their lives, how much time to allow for this resolution, and what future impact the problem may have. For example, a client who has been diagnosed with ulcerative colitis might be told, "Mr. Olson, the results of all our tests show that you have ulcerative colitis. We do not understand the cause of this illness, but there are no indications that any serious damage has occurred at this time. With proper treatment and medication, we should be able to keep active flare-ups at a minimum and prevent further complications."

The interview might continue at this point with a discussion of the client's lifestyle. Continue the discussion with ways to help the client cope with the impact of this disease and a description of the treatment necessary.

It might also continue as follows: "There is no cure for this disease and you may have many exacerbations and remissions throughout your life, but if this treatment works, there should be no complicating medical problems. However, it is important for us to treat this problem now, because if untreated, it can become serious. It is a good idea for you to include more fiber in your diet. I have a suggested nutritional plan here for you to consider. If certain foods cause diarrhea, then eliminate them from your diet or do not eat them during an active flare-up. In the active stage of this disease, avoid excess stress as much as possible. Also, I have a prescription to give you to assist the healing process in your lower colon, and medication to help prevent complications. You should see an improvement within several days."

Allow time for the client to think about what has just been said and to formulate any questions that arise. This is a good time to fill out the prescription or to get the nutritional guidelines from your file. Even saying "You must have some questions now, too" can be helpful to the client. If there are no questions at this point, remind the client, "Remember to call or email me any time you have a question. If you have any concerns or you are not better in a few days, call me. At any rate, I will want to see you again in six weeks to make certain that we are on the right track."

It is most helpful to write out instructions for clients or to provide them with some written material explaining the procedures they are to follow. The best medical advice can be lost if clients do not correctly follow instructions.

It cannot be emphasized enough that the helping interview will either be the key to a health care professional's success or be the end of what might have been a therapeutic relationship. Recall the incident identified in Chapter 1 (see p. 3) with Mrs. Nelson, who had been seriously injured by a dog. Consider how different the outcome might have been had her PCP been more "in tune" with her needs during the interview.

Case Study: Mrs. Nelson Revisited

When Mrs. Nelson called her primary care provider, it would have been much more therapeutic had the assistant said, "Oh, Mrs. Nelson, how awful. You say the emergency room physician asked that you have a blood test this morning and that you have his records with you? We usually only see patients receiving complete physicals in the morning, but I believe that the doctor will want to comply with the emergency room physician. Would you mind if you had to wait a bit when you come in?"

Mrs. Nelson, who has already shown that she is a compliant client, responds in the affirmative and the assistant selects a time where the wait will be as minimal as possible. When she is ushered into an examination room and blood has been taken, the doctor might have said, "My assistant tells me you had a frightening experience with a dog, Mrs. Nelson. Tell me what happened."

While the doctor listens and observes Mrs. Nelson, he will notice her bandaged head and finger and how uncomfortable she appears. It is likely that questions will be asked of Mrs. Nelson regarding the medical chart from the emergency room to further enhance her provider's record. It seems important, also, for the doctor to say, "May I remove your bandage to have a look at your injury while the assistant is checking your blood count for us?"

Both head and finger wounds are examined and appropriately bandaged by the doctor. Throughout this process, and a discussion of the fractured tailbone and ways to be more comfortable, Mrs. Nelson is still showing anxiety. The doctor might then say,

"You seem quite anxious and worried, Mrs. Nelson."

"Well, I am, I guess. This is a heck of a spot to be in. I love dogs so much; to think I could be attacked by one! If I lose my little poodle, I will be really mad. And you know, my husband and I are about to celebrate our 52nd wedding anniversary. We usually go someplace. I guess I won't be doing that, will I?"

"It is pretty hard to see a dog attack your dog and get hurt in the meantime, I know. I have a dog, and I think I would feel awful if something like that happened to her, especially when she did nothing to provoke the attack. How is your poodle?"

"Well, the vet says he will make it, but he looks awful. My husband picked him up at the vet this morning."

"As for going somewhere, you should still be able to go. You can remove this bandage tomorrow and come back in two days so I can remove the stitches. Then get yourself to the hair salon and they will be able to cover up the part of your head that was shaved. Your finger can be put into a more comfortable splint in a couple of days, too. The fractured tailbone is going to cause you the most problem for a while, so it might be good to get away where you won't have the responsibilities of all your household chores. Let someone else do all your cooking and cleaning. Traveling with a comfortable pillow to sit on is the only suggestion I might make to you."

"But what in the world will I do in the meantime? Look at all the dried blood still matted in my hair. This is awful."

"My assistant will be able to get a lot of that out for you. The rest will have to wait until the stitches are removed. Then you can have it shampooed."

"What a relief that would be. Maybe we can still take a little trip. Maybe even our poodle will be well enough to be gone for a while, too. I'm certain I'll need some information from you for the dog-owner's insurance. Will I be able to get that?"

"You call me and I'll be glad to supply anything that is required. Let me know if you have any problems with your injuries. I see that you are scheduled for your annual physical soon. Let's set that appointment for the first part of next month so we can check everything again for you."

Mrs. Nelson leaves the clinic with her hair a little cleaner, reassurances from her provider, recognition of the trauma she had been through, and another appointment. The therapeutic relationship will continue.

Case Study   *(Continued)*

Stop and Consider   4.3

Refer to Appendix A (see p. 278) and Maslow's Hierarchy of Needs.

1. Can you identify how and when the provider in this example elevated Mrs. Nelson's hierarchy of needs?

2. In what level of need did the conversation begin?

3. In what level of need did it end?

4. How does Maslow's Hierarchy of Needs relate to those needs identified in Welter's levels of needs?

SUMMARY

The helping interview is a critical component of any therapeutic helping relationship. First impressions are very important, and last much longer than any care that is given to clients. Every action, every word, every experience is imprinted upon the participating client, who will experience either a positive or a negative reaction to the process. Health care professionals who perform this interview many times daily are to be constantly reminded that this is the first time for their client, and that their full attention is required. Giving full attention means that the health care professional sets aside any personal agenda to make certain that the client's needs are met and that necessary information is gained.

EXERCISES

Exercise 1

Professional

The following paragraph identifies personal appearance appropriate for health care professionals. Do you agree or disagree? Explain your rationale. Recall a negative and a positive experience with a health care professional that was reflected by that professional's personal appearance.

A daily bath, an effective deodorant, and fresh breath are essential personal characteristics. Hair that is clean, off the collar, and out of the face is both sanitary and easy to care for. Even the most attractive hair should not be on the collar while at work. Nails should be trimmed and neatly manicured. Any polish worn should be clear only. Hands must be washed or sanitized after introduction to clients. Any uniform worn should fit properly and be appropriate for the setting. No aftershave or cologne should be worn. Men who are clean-shaven may be more acceptable to some clients than those with beards. It is best to wear no jewelry, with the exception of post earrings and wedding bands. Multiple body piercings and tattoos are offensive to many clients; therefore, they should be eliminated or kept covered whenever possible.

Exercise 2

Consider what your response might be to the following client statements made in the interview process.

1. "I want my sister to come in with me for the examination."
   Response _____

2. "Yeah, those are my meds, but I stopped taking the little green ones because they upset my stomach."
   Response _____

3. "Why do I have to get on the scale every time I come here? It is embarrassing."
   Response _____

4. "You're not going to have to give my little guy a shot, are you?"
   Response _____

5. "Why won't you tell me the test results? Why do I have to wait for the doctor?"
   Response _____

6. "My best friend died of a heart attack this year. Can you do an EKG just to make sure everything is okay?"
   Response _____

7. "My wife made me come for this physical exam; otherwise, I wouldn't be here."
   Response _____

Exercise 3

1. Keep a journal every day for a week. In this journal, be aware of just one person who might have a problem. Can you identify the level of need? How about your own problems? Can you identify the levels of need and the helping responses?

2. Be aware of roadblocks to communication that you create or that you observe in other conversations. Make a note of these in your journal and identify how the roadblock could be changed to a helping response.

To be successful in these exercises, you will probably need to review daily the material in this chapter that identifies levels of need and roadblocks.

Exercise 4

Identify the following as closed or open-ended questions, indirect statements, or roadblocks.

1. _____ How are you feeling today?

2. _____ You're looking pretty chipper today.

3. _____ Why did you do that?

4. _____ When I lift your leg, does it hurt?

5. _____ Oh, don't worry; everything will be fine.

6. _____ You're not getting old.

7. _____ Oh, it couldn't possibly feel like that.

8. _____ You say the accident happened this morning?

9. _____ What did the doctor tell you about the test results?

10. _____ Tell me about the test results.

11. _____ Could you tell me when you think this started?

12. _____ I'd like to hear about your new job.

13. _____ Why do you think you feel this way?

REVIEW QUESTIONS

Multiple Choice

1. What are the three components of the helping interview?

   a. Greeting, identifying client's problem, and the professional's visit

   b. Orientation of each other, identifying the problem, and resolution of problem

   c. Open communication, hearing the problem, and clinic follow-up

   d. Orientation, open communication, and resolution of problem

2. The orientation phase of the helping interview should find the health care professional using which of the following skills?

   a. Sharing observations, acknowledging feelings, clarifying and validating, reflecting and paraphrasing

   b. Giving advice, requiring explanations, seeking approval, correcting, and defending

   c. Showing warmth, being genuine, establishing trust, and expressing sympathy/empathy and sincerity

   d. Introducing client to the clinic, reviewing client's medical chart, discussing billing procedures, and monitoring insurance claims

3. Which statement describes an indirect statement?

   a. Does not require the client to enlarge upon the response.

   b. Can usually be answered with a *yes* or a *no*.

   c. Encourages clients to identify more of the problem.

   d. Calls for a client response without the client feeling questioned.

4. With today's changes in health care, which of the following is important?

   a. Empower the client to actively participate in his or her health care.

   b. Maintain the same health care provider through the adult years.

   c. Pay close attention to television ads for drugs and medicines.

   d. Have clients pay as much of their health care costs as possible.

5. When conducting the helping interview, what is best for the health care professional to do?

   a. Have the client sit on the examination table.

   b. Address the client informally to ease his/her anxiety.

   c. Have the client not disrobe during the interview orientation.

   d. Dress casually yourself so the client is not intimidated.

FOR FURTHER CONSIDERATION

1. With another person in your class, identify ways in which the orientation phase of the helping interview with James Alonzo (from the opening case study) could be more productive and provide better care management. Once you have identified the changes you would make, role-play the orientation for your class.

2. What action might be taken to reduce James Alonzo's dislike of seeing a doctor and having a physical examination? How might the medical assistant encourage him?

3. Gather as much information as you can about what medically oriented Web sites are most reputable and why. What questions would you ask yourself before relying upon a particular site? What kind of information can you share with clients who regularly use the Internet for information? Identify the particular sites you would recommend and justify your choices.

CASE STUDIES

Case Study 1

Alice Jameson is a 69-year-old who has been suffering from flu-like symptoms for several days. She calls her primary care provider to make an appointment. This conversation follows:

"Mid-Town Medical Clinic, this is Marianne; please hold." After a 2- to 3-minute wait, the receptionist comes back on the line.

"Thank you for holding. Can I help you?"

"This is Alice Jameson. I am feeling terrible. I think I have the flu. But I shouldn't have the flu; I got the flu shot last fall. Can I see my doctor?"

"Alice, we are so busy with flu patients, I don't have an opening until day after tomorrow. Can you come at 3:30 P.M.?"

After a brief pause, Alice responds, hesitantly.

"No, I don't think so. If I don't get better, I guess I'll go to my neighborhood emergency care clinic."

"Okay. Bye."

The receptionist at Mid-Town Medical Clinic does not learn that Alice has had a fever of 101 degrees for 2 days and does not recall that she had surgery to place an artificial heart valve just 8 months ago.

1. Identify Alice's need. Were those needs met?

2. Name the problems that exist in this situation.

3. Role-play a helping interview that can be therapeutic *and* can meet Alice's needs. Assume that the clinic's schedule really is full.

Case Study 2

At the close of a presurgical examination, it is your responsibility to bring the client written instructions related to hospital admission and presurgery preparations. As you present the information to Mia Trong, you sense that she may still have some questions. She seems hesitant to leave.

1. What will you say? What will you do?

2. What steps do you take to make certain Mia's questions have all been addressed?

REFERENCES AND RESOURCES

Brammer, L. M., & MacDonald, G. (2002). *The helping relationship: Process and skills* (8th ed.). Boston: Allyn & Bacon.

Desmond, J., & Copeland, L. R. (2000). *Communicating with today's patient*. San Francisco: Jossey-Bass.

Libster, M. (2001). *Demonstrating care: The art of integrative nursing*. Albany, NY: Thomson Delmar Learning.

van Servellen, G. (2009). *Communication skills for the health care professional: Concepts, practice, and evidence*. Sudbury, MA: Jones & Bartlett.

Welter, P. (1990). *How to help a friend*. Wheaton, IL: Tyndale House.

Chapter 5
The Therapeutic Response across the Life Span

CHAPTER OBJECTIVES

After completing this chapter, the learner should be able to:

- Define the key terms as presented in the glossary.

- Describe popular theories of human growth and development and identify the various stages found in Appendix A (pp. 268–287).

- Discuss appropriate methods health care professionals might use to encourage a healthy lifestyle as part of moral development.

- Recall a minimum of five characteristics each that are particular to infants, children, adolescents, adults, and older adults.

- List at least four guidelines for therapeutic communication for each age group, giving an example of how each might be instituted.

- Discuss the concept that, to be truly therapeutic, health care professionals must genuinely like their work and the age groups they are treating.

Opening Case Study

Dr. Charles Lewien, CEO of a large family practice clinic, was preparing a seminar for presentation to staff members on the subject of how to improve client communication. While musing on these thoughts, he was surprised by the circular nature of the life span encompassed by the clients seen at the clinic. Infants are totally dependent on caregivers and communicate by reactions to discomfort and pain and by touch. Children can vocalize but are very present focused, and often fearful. These behaviors require communication at a low level of understanding. Adolescents present a wall, separating them from all adults, and vary from behaving as a child one moment and as an adult the next. Adults would seem to be the easiest to communicate with, but they are frequently blindsided by their own concerns with raising a family, careers, and sexuality, making communication difficult. Older adults bring the communication challenge full circle, as they become less independent, losing cognitive ability and experiencing decreasing mental sharpness. Dr. Lewien pondered whether any communication techniques are consistently applicable to each age group.

Stop and Consider 5.1

1. Which age groups have you communicated with and what have you observed?

2. Were you able to consistently apply any particular therapeutic communication techniques to each age group? Why or why not?

INTRODUCTION

Professionalism

The health care professional should have a sound background in and understanding of biological human growth and development, and must, of necessity, consider these principles when communicating with others.

To communicate therapeutically, helping professionals must also consider a person's lifetime experiences, conditioning, predisposition and inherited characteristics, life cycle and life span, relationship to others, learning abilities and vocation, and cultural background.

Many prominent theories of human growth and development and psychology exist. Of all the theories known, no *one* theory is generally accepted. Perhaps this is because, as Carl Rogers, the psychotherapist, believes, we are still in process. We are still learning and developing more viable and creative ways to live and work.

The goal of any health care professional is to enable individuals to get in touch with themselves, to encourage them to discover a full and functioning life with meaning and purpose. Therefore, the more health care professionals know and understand about human growth and development, the better prepared they will be to offer therapeutic communication.

In the opening case study, Dr. Lewien makes the point that communication is greatly influenced by age and follows a continuous loop of behavior. In the infant stage, communication is totally nonverbal, involving the senses and body language. Children and adolescents communicate with age increasing language sophistication and complexity combined with a time focus ranging from present to future. Adults reverse this pattern, going from complex sophisticated language and a future time focus to simple language and present time focus. The senses play a lesser role with older adults as eyesight, hearing, and sometimes smell and touch diminish. The complexity of communication channels associated with age has important implications for health care providers, making therapeutic communication more challenging.

In addition to the information presented in this chapter, a review of Appendix A: Theories of Growth and Development (pp. 268–287) will be helpful in learning more about growth and development throughout the life span.

INFANTS

Case Study: Infants

John and Hannah Adams have had their first child, a son, home from the hospital just 3 days. John calls the pediatrician because he is worried about circumcision care. He noticed the formation of a yellow crust on the penis. Their son had a Gomco circumcision prior to leaving the hospital. The pediatrician reassures John that the crusted exudate is commonly seen on the glans penis and is normal and often observed during the healing process. The Adamses are encouraged to express any future concerns and to continue the good care of their son.

The preceding case study illustrates the therapeutic response to the infant caregiver: the medical professional explains the normal healing process and encourages the Adamses to continue the good care of their son and to feel free to call with any other health concerns. If the infant communicates discomfort by crying or being fussy, checking for signs of infection may be necessary. Infants are totally dependent upon their caregivers and have limited means of communicating their needs.

The infant stage of growth and development is very rapid and covers the time period from birth to 1 year of age (Figure 5-1). During infancy, the child is totally dependent upon parents and caregivers. Physical comfort and safety are primary considerations during this phase of growth, since infants cannot communicate their needs with spoken words. They may cry because a wet or messy diaper is uncomfortable, or because they are hungry or in pain. As the infant develops they may learn they receive attention from others when they cry.

In an effort to communicate more effectively with their infants, some parents begin teaching sign language at 6–7 months of age. Many infants begin to sign back between 8 and 9 months simple signs such as "more," "all done," and "milk." Signing enables the child to communicate long before they can vocalize actual words and can reduce stress for the child and their parents and caregivers. Some infants can sign 12 or more signs at 12 months and by 18 months have a signing vocabulary of nearly 100 words and phrases.

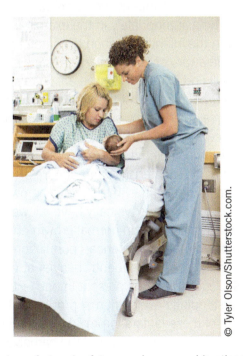

© Tyler Olson/Shutterstock.com.

FIGURE 5-1   Physical comfort and safety are primary considerations during infancy.

The Therapeutic Response

A therapeutic response to the infant consists of close observation and touch, which enhances the bonding process between the caregiver and infant and stimulates the infant.

Safety issues should be a primary concern. Infants can easily roll off tables and counters, so never take your eyes or hands off them. Observe what is within reach of infants, and prevent them from grabbing or kicking items that could be a hazard.

Infants should be held lovingly for a few minutes on each visit, and especially after every painful procedure. They are sensitive to touch and need warmth and love. Holding them will help the infant associate the health care professional with feelings other than pain.

At about 3 months, infants begin to recognize familiar faces and voices. When possible, include the parent or caregiver in procedures as security for the infant. Speaking in a soft, calm voice reassures the infant and caregiver.

Create an environment that is pleasant for the infant. At 8 months, the infant is developing a memory. Wearing colorful uniform tops or jackets or large buttons for interest helps create a comfortable atmosphere. Mobiles hung appropriately in the examination room add interest and may divert the infant's attention to something pleasurable.

Cultural

⊕ *Be aware of family characteristics and culture.* Medical professionals will find it helpful to have an *understanding* of the ethnic, cultural, and family background of the infant. Some cultures and religions may not endorse any circumcision while others may follow specific age-related times or ceremonial rituals for circumcision. Other families opt to have circumcision completed before leaving the hospital or a few days after birth. Family characteristics and culture also influence the interpretation of apparent irregularities in the infant's growth and development. For example, Asian infants typically have a lower birth weight and are shorter than the lengths given on normal growth charts, which are biased toward the majority European American population. In similar fashion, Native American infants are frequently heavier at birth than European American infants. Genetic patterns present in one or both parents can be critical to understanding developmental problems. Medical professionals must be aware of these factors to provide the necessary therapeutic response beneficial to both the infant and the caregiver.

Parents and caregivers often have questions about infant care. Take the time to listen carefully to their questions and concerns. Restate the question or concern to validate and clarify that you have heard correctly. Respond to each query by providing information, instructing, or demonstrating procedures to educate the parent or caregiver.

Stop and Consider 5.2

Reread the infant case study and respond to the following questions.

1. What questions might be asked to assess the infant's health status?

2. How was the pediatrician therapeutic in response to John's concerns?

3. How does the case study reflect B. F. Skinner's theory of operant conditioning described in Appendix A?

CHILDREN

Case Study: Children

Katie is going to the doctor today. She is 2½ years old and is excited about going because they have such great toys for her to play with. When she arrives with her grandma, she goes straight for the toys. The wait is not long; when the medical assistant is ready, she calls Katie by name. In the examination room, the provider talks directly to Katie, and allows her to play with the stethoscope and to listen to her heartbeat. Katie is not afraid because she likes the provider (Figure 5-2).

Any person may have difficulty adjusting to being ill and to being under the care of a health care provider. Children may have an even more difficult time because they do not fully understand what is happening to them. Children cannot comprehend why the medicine or treatment is going to help them feel better. Some children even feel they are being punished or have done something terribly wrong when they are ill.

Children, like all human beings, fear what they do not know or understand. Even the smallest procedure seems major. Parents, primary caregivers, and health care professionals who take the time to explain what is

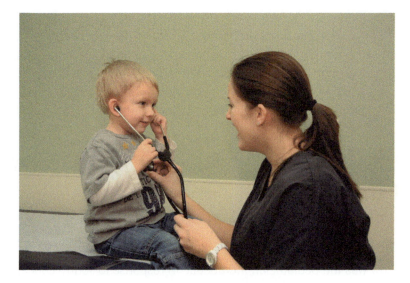

FIGURE 5-2   Focusing your attention on the child and making eye contact at his or her level are ways to be therapeutic.

happening and to increase a child's knowledge are apt to have a soothing effect and reduce their anxiety. Having a consistent routine during visits allows the children to anticipate what to expect and reduces their fear.

A health care professional will want to consider the relationship between children and the parents or primary caregivers. A good relationship with caregivers will lessen any problems with their children.

The Therapeutic Response

The environment is important for children. Pediatric clinics should be colorful, attractive, and comfortable. There should be safe and clean toys to keep their minds active and distracted from procedures.

The health care professional should establish a friendly relationship with each child. This is accomplished by focusing attention on the child. Kneel in front of them, make eye contact, and speak directly to them on their level of understanding. Mention something positive about the shirt or shoes they are wearing or ask something about the teddy bear they are holding. A positive approach, praise for accomplishments, and acknowledgment of desirable behaviors is much more effective than negative or critical approaches.

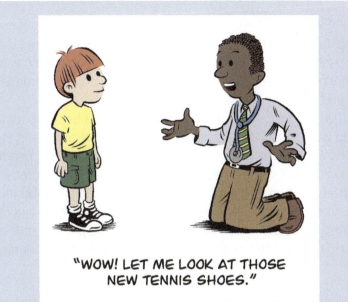

"WOW! LET ME LOOK AT THOSE
NEW TENNIS SHOES."

Give a child a choice only when you know the decision will be the correct one. For example, "Shall we see how tall you are first or how much you weigh?" It makes no difference which choice is made; both procedures will be accomplished. Let children help with procedures if you can, but do not lose control of the situation. Johnny may hold the tape while you apply the bandage to his leg.

Do not keep children and their parents waiting. Children become anxious quickly. Visits to the clinic that are short, have some pleasant experiences, and have friendly, caring health care professionals whom children recognize are the most effective visits.

Help children deal with their feelings. When children ask questions, respond in short, simple answers. Be truthful and honest. Children who become angry and frustrated can hit a doll, pound clay, or draw pictures. Health care professionals should not expect to be rewarded by children for the examination, especially if it involves anything painful. In fact, children may tell you they do not like you.

Listen to the feelings children express, verbally or nonverbally. Learn as much about pediatric clients as possible from parents. Recognize that crying and silence are pleas for comfort and care as well as anger and frustration.

(continues)

The Therapeutic Response   (*Continued*)

Listen to parents' concerns. Respond truthfully, even if the facts may be upsetting. Help parents deal with their children's feelings and behavior. Encourage them to reinforce with warmth and tenderness rather than fear and anxiety.

Give rewards. They can be simple; a hug, a high-five, or a knuckle-bump is good. Children especially enjoy stickers and hand stamps.

 Be aware of your own feelings when approaching children. They know instantly if you are insecure or do not like them. Children can be "unlovable" when they are frustrated, angry, and in pain. You must be personally able to handle their feelings. Working with children is a challenge, but one that, fortunately, many dedicated health care professionals enjoy. Keep in mind these guidelines and remember to always enjoy your profession.

Self-Awareness

Stop and Consider 5.3

Review "Case Study: Children" and respond to the following questions.

1. Identify therapeutic responses or actions the medical assistant and the provider incorporated to help Katie feel more comfortable during her visit today.

2. Consult Appendix A to determine which of Piaget's cognitive development learning theories Katie is currently experiencing.

3. Why is it important to develop a consistent routine during clinic visits for this age group?

ADOLESCENTS

Case Study: Adolescents

Taking Jeff, age 14, to the pediatrician as a teenager was different from when he was younger. As they were driving to the clinic, Jeff's mom asked if he would prefer to see the provider alone. Jeff's immediate response was "Yes." His mom assured him that she was there if he needed her. When they arrived, Jeff quickly picked up one of the car magazines that the clinic staff had available and promptly ignored the two children playing in the child's corner.

When Jeff was called, he proudly marched to the examination room alone. During the examination, the provider posed a question that he always asked of teenagers: "Jeff, are you sexually active?" Jeff, a little embarrassed, responded negatively, but the provider hastened to go on. "It is a question I ask all my teenage clients, and I'll ask you when you are in next year. It is important for me to have a truthful answer. It is good you are not yet sexually active. Girls are wonderful; sex is wonderful; but both are addicting." Jeff laughed. The ice had been broken for future discussions regarding sex.

Adolescence is a period of transition from childhood to adulthood. Adolescents fight for their independence, yet have the same needs for comfort and security as children. It is a turbulent time for teenagers, as well as for their parents and primary caregivers.

Many demands are placed on adolescents. The demands come from family, school, peers, and society. The bodies of adolescents are changing. They are awkward and feel unsure of themselves. They are confused by their sexual feelings. It is a time when it is vitally important that the adolescents have something to feel good about.

The challenges adolescents face often seem insurmountable to them. They may suffer from unsightly acne. Many girls have painful menstruation. Boys may begin to have nocturnal emissions. There is an enormous amount of pressure from peers, who often have a misguided notion or fantasy of what an adolescent is expected to be.

Another reason this is a difficult period is that parents, who are often occupied with earning a living and making a career for themselves while supporting their families, are also perplexed with the sudden changes in their adolescent sons and daughters. Teenagers and their parents are likely to have opposing views on just about everything.

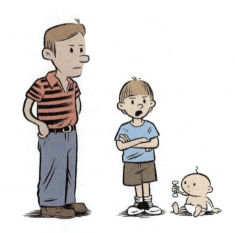

"WHY CAN'T I DRIVE?"

The Therapeutic Response

Allow the adolescent privacy and the right to be examined or treated without parents present. It is best not to moralize, but to generate an atmosphere in which the teenager will feel comfortable enough to ask questions and seek information.

Do not assume that parents have told their teenagers everything they need to know about sex. Use correct anatomical and socially accepted terms for genitalia and sexual expressions, and provide accurate and factual information through books, pamphlets, and videos. Not only do adolescents need to understand their sexuality physiologically and emotionally, they also must understand safe sex and the responsibility that goes with being sexually active. Health care professionals often avoid this topic, but events in today's society no longer allow such an attitude.

Treat adolescents with respect and dignity. Ask open-ended questions about their worries and concerns and avoid making comments about their clothes or hairstyle or speaking about good grades as the only important endeavor. Find out what is important in their lives, how they like to spend their time, and what kinds of concerns they have. Make notes in their medical record so you can bring up the topic at their next visit.

Set limits that are fair and consistent. Discourage antisocial behavior while encouraging self-control and establishment of identity. Do not take sides in a teenager's battle with parents. Help both parent and teenager assess and understand their positions.

 You must clearly like and care about adolescents. If you do not, you will be ineffective in being therapeutic. You cannot hide your feelings from children and adolescents.

Self-Awareness

Set the stage for the adolescents' transfer from pediatric care to adult care. Young adults often struggle in this transition to establish a relationship with a personal provider. During the college years or their first years of employment, young adults are often away from home and have only minimal financial resources. Help instill in their minds the importance of quality health care throughout their lifetime.

Adolescents need to feel a sense of worth. They need time and understanding to resolve the tensions they feel. The health care professional can be a positive force in this direction. Adolescents welcome established limits that offer security but allow them to gain a little bit of independence. Listen to the adolescent; you may be surprised at what you learn.

Stop and Consider 5.4

Recall the case study about Jeff's visit to the clinic and respond to the following questions.

1. How might it be different to take Jeff to the provider as a child compared to as an adolescent?

2. Review Freud's psychosexual stages of development as presented in Appendix A. Freud theorized that each individual's behavior consists of three major forces: the id, the ego, and the superego. Which force do you think is more prominent in Jeff's life as an adolescent?

3. Suppose Jeff were deaf. Would you do anything additional or change anything to ensure therapeutic communication?

ADULTS

Case Study: Adults

Karen, a 40-year-old mother, presents for her annual physical examination. As the assistant is recording Karen's vital signs and taking her medical history, she asks how everything else is going. Karen relates some difficulty dealing with a teenage daughter who is not doing well in school and whose behavior is troublesome. The assistant responds, "That is quite a worry, isn't it? Dr. Henley has a lot of skills in helping parents cope with teenagers. Let me mention your concern to him. Also, we have some wonderful pamphlets at the front desk that might help. I'll collect some for you to take home."

Karen is relieved that she will be able to talk with someone about her concerns. She has been feeling like such a failure as a parent.

Many of the principles applied to children and adolescents are appropriate for adults of all ages. Adults should be recognized for the characteristic activities of this age group—working toward career goals, earning a living, establishing primary relationships, making a place for themselves in a community, and perhaps raising a family.

Because these activities require an inordinate amount of time and responsibility, a fair amount of stress-related complaints will be found in this age group. This group can also benefit from information and assistance regarding daily living and parenting. For instance, if a child suffers from a chronic illness, the astute and therapeutic provider recognizes the need to also care for the parents. Education will be an important component of each helping interview.

Younger adults may actually be living in an extended psychological adolescent period, since many are still pursuing an education or are not independent from parents. Many young adults complete college and land their first job, but can't afford to live on their own. A fair number of young adults return home to live with mom and dad again. This age group has been termed the "boomerang generation." The fact that these young adults are physically mature and are most likely living an adult life in all other ways is a source of conflict to be recognized.

Physically, persons in this age group are quite healthy. Women are apt to be bearing children in the younger adult years or facing menopause in their 40s and 50s. Men will pass through a period identified as climacteric, when their hormone production tends to slow and diminish.

The Therapeutic Response

It is especially crucial during the adult years to recognize the unequal partnership occurring between client and provider and to equalize the relationship as much as possible. Keep the following therapeutic recommendations in mind.

Get to know adult clients. Never allow a therapeutic interview to pass without a discussion of what is happening in the client's life. As much care will be given with an honest discussion of daily occurrences as from a discussion of a particular ailment or chief complaint.

Cultural

⊕ *Be aware and sensitive to the cultures, lifestyles, and religious beliefs of clients.* Cultural variations regarding personal space, physical touch, eye contact, hand gestures, etc. vary from one culture to another. If you are not sure of cultural etiquette, discuss it with the client. Observe their actions and follow their lead.

Recognize the skills and intelligence of clients and do not try to impress them by unnecessary use of medical nomenclature. Explain health issues in terms clients will understand and comprehend. Do not talk down to clients. Recognize the client's desire for information and knowledge regarding treatment and care.

Emphasize preventive health care. While most adults see the provider for a "cure" or treatment for an ailment, use that opportunity to educate clients regarding preventative health measures. This is the life stage when prevention can save time and money and lead to better health in the later adult years (Figure 5-3).

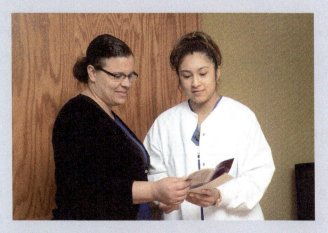

FIGURE 5-3   Health care professionals will want to emphasize preventative health care to adults.

Recognize your role as a member of the health care team. Adults are likely to have more than one primary care provider. Consider the woman who receives care during pregnancy and delivery from an OB/GYN and staff, but still sees a family provider for all other care. This duplication should complement rather than conflict.

Recognize the stress caused by any accident or serious illness in this age group. This is the age identified as the "prime of life." Any serious ailment or accident is apt to be met with anger, denial, and depression. People in this age group do not think about death or disability; they put off such thoughts for the later adult years.

Legal

Respect clients' right to privacy. Clients have a right to expect that the information shared with health care professionals is protected. Adults often reveal information that could compromise their reputation if known to others. Confidentiality must always be preserved and is mandated by HIPAA.

Encourage adult clients to hope for the best, but do not promise specific results. Health care professionals cannot predict a sure outcome and should never do so. Promising a cure only destroys the therapeutic relationship if or when the cure does not occur.

Stop and Consider 5.5

Review the adult case study, and then respond to the following questions.

1. Review Erikson's stages of psychosocial development in Appendix A. Which of Erikson's psychosocial stages of development is Karen in at the present time?

2. Do you think the assistant responded appropriately to Karen's comments about her daughter? Justify your answer.

OLDER ADULTS

Case Study: Older Adults

Mr. Levine is 78 years of age. He has just learned that he has prostate cancer and must have radiation treatment. He is confused about what all this means. Using an anatomical picture, the provider shows Mr. Levine where the cancer is located. He tells him that the good news is that the examination showed the cancer was not advanced, nor had it spread.

Treatment is detailed carefully. Mr. Levine asks the provider to write some of this down so he will be able to tell his daughter what is happening. The provider complies and tells him what to expect from the treatment. The medical assistant verifies that Mr. Levine still lives with his daughter and that she has medical power of attorney as documented in his medical records. Mr. Levine leaves the clinic with an appointment to see a radiologist, and is told to feel free to call any time with any questions or concerns.

Older adults experience fewer acute illnesses. However, chronic illnesses, such as hypertension, diabetes, arthritis, and hearing and vision impairment, often plague this age group. At the same time, a loss of self-identity and feelings of belonging often occur when a person retires and/or experiences lifestyle changes.

Older adults may look forward to this period as a time of more freedom, a time to pursue activities they never accomplished in their younger years, and a time of fewer obligations. Others may look at this final stage as a time when they no longer feel needed, a time when they become bored and lack the energy to participate in new activities, and a time of fear for the loss of personal safety, financial security, and good health.

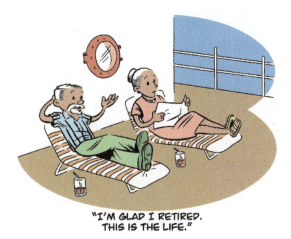

"I'M GLAD I RETIRED.
THIS IS THE LIFE."

The way younger years have been spent is likely the same way the later years will be spent. If a person has been active and involved, has been a member of one or more organizations, and has had many friends, the same activities usually continue. The individual who preferred to be alone, had few interests, and was not a member of any organization generally prefers the same lifestyle in later years. Some, especially those in business for themselves, find retirement difficult if they have no hobbies or interests. Illness, loss of a loved one, or relocation can disrupt lifestyle patterns and result in depression or withdrawal.

The 2010 Census Bureau reports that the number of people age 85 and older has increased to more than 1.9 million. This number is projected to quadruple over the next four decades. The number of people reaching age 65, along with their increased life expectancy, have caused the creation of three new age classifications. They are "young-old," 65–74 years of age; "old," 74–84 years of age; and "oldest-old," 85-plus years of age. The growing number of centenarians, 100-plus years of age, has doubled each decade since 1950 in most developed countries.

Many older adults are still living productive lives. For example a 90-year-old just recertified her CPR credential and continues to work 3 days a week as an operating room nurse. Another, 108 years old, threw the opening pitch for a Mariners baseball game recently. Older adults are living longer but do require specialized consideration. Consider the loss that many in this life stage experience: loss of a productive career; loss of a spouse or partner and friends; their children possibly preceding them in death; and loss of health, wealth, and autonomy. Some may lose the ability to keep their mental **cognition** and judgment. Greater health care options will be required to accommodate these growing numbers.

The Therapeutic Response

Self-Awareness

All of the therapeutic responses mentioned for the adult population should be followed for older adults as well. Some additional guidelines are appropriate. There is a tendency to stereotype older adults and at times to patronize them. Self-awareness regarding your personal feelings toward older adults will be crucial to therapeutic communication.

Allow additional time for older adults to compensate for physiological changes. This client requires more time to ambulate or to disrobe or dress, and may need assistance. More care should be taken in explaining procedures. Talk slowly and clearly. Allow for any sensory deprivation and do not be afraid to raise questions regarding a sensory loss to assess how a client might be better treated. Some are too embarrassed to ask about a hearing loss, for instance, but are relieved when a provider discusses it.

During face-to-face communication with older adult clients, minimize background noise, face them when speaking, and use visual aids to help clarify and reinforce understanding of any key points.

Comfort is important at this age. Be sure the reception room furniture is comfortable. It is easier for older clients to rise from a firm, straight-backed chair with arms than from a soft, low sofa. Assess whether the examination rooms are adaptable to older adults. Provide pillows for support and comfort. Handrails in the restroom provide security and support and allow older adults freedom to be autonomous. Remember, many older adults are very sensitive to touch and arthritis may be painful. When caring for older adults, be aware of their pain level and use a gentle touch (Figure 5-4).

A set schedule is often best. Older adults are comfortable and secure in a routine. Allow for that routine. If a person must be seen weekly to monitor blood pressure, ask that they come in on the same day at the same time each week.

Older persons are to be treated with respect and with the recognition that their lives are valuable. Do not operate under the assumption that "since you've lived a full life, you probably won't want to…." Treatment is as important to older adults as it is to youth.

Do not be over solicitous or overprotective. This only serves to reduce self-esteem and intensify the feelings older adults may be having. Verbal and nonverbal communication can help the client retain self-esteem and confidence during the later years. Ask what the client's likes and dislikes are about the clinic and his or her care.

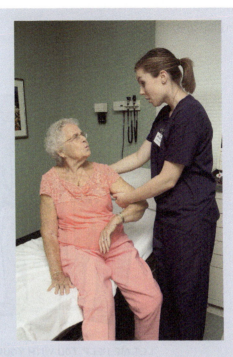

FIGURE 5-4   Minute pressure can be uncomfortable, even painful, for the older adult.

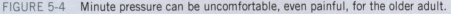

Cultural

⊕ *Inquire about cultural and religious beliefs and values pertaining to illness and death.* As much as possible, incorporate these preferences into the clients' treatment plan if they do not contraindicate. Many clinics encourage older clients to complete directives for end-of-life choices.

Interest older adult clients in activities as much as possible. A discussion of their daily activities helps to assess if they might benefit from additional activity in their lives. In making suggestions, consider their aptitude, physical abilities, and interests. Be aware of appropriate referrals, such as adult daycare, senior citizens' centers and Medicare's Silver Sneaker program.

Help the older adult clients remain independent as long as possible. However, do not be afraid to honestly indicate when it is time for additional care or altered living situations. Talking with clients to determine what kind of plans they have for the time when they can no longer adequately care for themselves is beneficial in helping clients make their own decisions.

(continues)

The Therapeutic Response   (*Continued*)

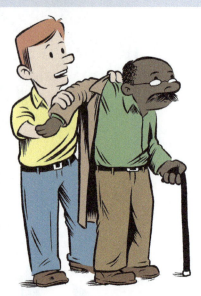

"LET ME HELP YOU WITH YOUR COAT."

Remember the needs of the primary caregivers of the older adult. Whether caring for the older adult in an "at-home" environment or in one of the many institutional facilities available today, primary caregivers must have a respite. A weekend or even a day free of caregiving responsibility is revitalizing and necessary for all parties concerned.

Self-Awareness

Understand your own feelings toward aging parents or growing older yourself. Try to determine how you would like to be treated and provide the same courtesy to your older clients. The entire staff has the responsibility of helping older adults feel needed and wanted.

Remember that some diseases/disorders may affect cognition. Cognition refers to processes by which a person knows the world and interacts with it. Cognition involves the way in which the brain learns and interprets information. The human brain is a very delicate and sensitive organ that is susceptible to injury from both internal and external factors. Falls causing blows to the head are an example of internal factors that may result in brain injury. The use and/or side effects of some drugs, electrolyte imbalance, and ischemia caused by some disease processes are examples of external factors affecting brain function. Therapeutic responses must allow for the cognitive aspect.

Stop and Consider 5.6

Review "Case Study: Older Adults" and respond to the following questions.

1. Identify therapeutic responses or actions the provider incorporated to help Mr. Levine understand his health care problem and treatment plan.

2. Consult Appendix A to determine which of Erikson's eight psychosocial crises Mr. Levine is progressing through.

3. What other therapeutic responses and/or actions are important to remember when working with this age group?

SUMMARY

Understanding human growth and development is essential for health care professionals if they are to communicate effectively with their clients. Lifetime experiences, education, predisposition and inherited characteristics, as well as culture, lifestyle, and religion are important factors to be considered. The more health care professionals know and understand growth and development, the better prepared they will be to offer therapeutic responses. Therapeutic communication should be aimed toward helping clients get in touch with themselves and encouraging them to discover a full and functioning life with meaning and purpose.

Professionalism

One of the concepts identified throughout the various age groups is the idea that, to be effective in therapeutic communication, health care professionals must genuinely like their work and the age groups they are treating. Having a healthy respect for life and for each age group and its particular challenges and a mature notion regarding dying and death is a must for effective therapeutic communications. Table 5-1 provides a summary of typical characteristics across the life span.

TABLE 5-1   **Brief Summary of Characteristics across the Life span**

Age Group	Characteristics	Therapeutic Considerations
Infant (birth to 1 year)	• Present focus • Communicates by crying and fussing • Responds to facial expression	• Ensure safety • Educate and instruct caregiver • Provide physical comfort and basic needs

(continues)

TABLE 5-1   Brief Summary of Characteristics across the Life span (*Continued*)

Age Group	Characteristics	Therapeutic Considerations
Child (1–12 years)	• Present focus • Little language sophistication • Body language • Responsible for own actions • Accepts authority outside home	• Speak at child's level of understanding • Empower by giving choices • Give rewards
Adolescent (13–21 years)	• Present to future focused • Changing body • Sexual awareness	• Allow privacy • Acknowledge period of transition • Set limits, be consistent
Adult (21–65+ years)	• Future focus • Sophisticated and complex language • Body language significant • Family and career oriented	• Support equal partnership with medical personnel • Be sensitive to cultures, lifestyles, and religion • Emphasize preventative medicine
Older adult (65–100+ years)	• Present focused • Decreasing language sophistication • Hearing and vision impairment • Possible loss of self-identity • Financial worries	• Compensate for physiological changes • Eliminate background noise, speak slower, use visual aids

EXERCISES

Exercise 1

In groups of three, identify your personal worst experience in a health care setting. Role-play with a group member how that situation could be turned from your worst experience into one that was therapeutic. Have the third person judge the therapeutic response.

Continue role-playing until each of you has shared a worst experience and identified how to make it therapeutic.

Exercise 2

Interview an older adult, an adolescent, and an adult. Ask the following questions:

1. When you last visited your provider, how were you treated?

2. What did you like the best?

3. What did you dislike?

4. Why do you seek care from this particular provider?

Exercise 3

Search the Internet for information about one or more of the age groups discussed in this chapter. Print out or prepare a list of the following:

- Telephone numbers and addresses that you might contact for literature.

- Internet sites, books, videos, or other media that age groups discussed in this chapter might be interested in researching.

- Resources for families needing support information for these age groups.

- Government Web sites for information on seniors' health care, Medicaid, Medicare, and support groups.

REVIEW QUESTIONS

Multiple Choice

1. What was Piaget's theory termed?
   a. Cognitive development
   b. Psychosexual stages of development
   c. Humanistic psychology
   d. Psychosocial crises

2. What is Sigmund Freud's *id* also known as?
   a. The ego
   b. The superego
   c. The pleasure principle
   d. The reality principle

3. Which behavioral learning theorist applies classical conditioning?
   a. Jean Piaget
   b. Lawrence Kohlberg
   c. Erik Erikson
   d. Ivan Pavlov

4. What is the premise of Erik Erikson's stages of growth and development termed?
   a. The reality principle
   b. The pleasure principle
   c. Psychosocial crises
   d. Stages of moral development

5. According to Piaget's stages of cognitive development, the child does not differentiate between self and other objects. The child repeats rewarding activities, discovers new ways to get what he or she wants, and may have imaginary friends. Which period is described?
   a. Sensorimotor period
   b. Concrete operations
   c. Preoperational period
   d. Autonomy versus shame and doubt

6. Which age group is described by the following statement? Reflection on and acceptance of one's life, feeling fulfilled, looking back on lives and accomplishments.
   a. Infants
   b. Adolescents
   c. Older adults
   d. Adults

7. Which age group is described? Demands come from family, school, peers, and society; still have needs for comfort and security; experiencing body changes and may be awkward; very modest.
   a. Older adults
   b. Adolescents
   c. Children
   d. Adults

8. Which statement regarding adolescents would be considered inappropriate?
   a. Adolescents fight for their independence, yet have the same needs for comfort and security as children.
   b. Health care professionals are often called upon to discuss a healthy lifestyle for teens.
   c. Adolescents should be treated with respect and dignity.
   d. Modesty and privacy are not important to adolescents.

9. Mr. Valdez, age 80, is being seen today for a follow-up appointment. Mr. Valdez is treasurer of the homeowners' association where he lives and is active in the community. Which of the following statements is not therapeutic?

   a. All older adults are considered senile and unable to live independently.

   b. Allow additional time to compensate for physiological changes.

   c. Address older adults using their full name and title to show respect.

   d. A set schedule is best for older adults.

10. Which theorist believes that individuals move back and forth from one need to another depending on the circumstances present at the time?

   a. Lawrence Kohlberg   **c.** Abraham Maslow

   b. Jean Piaget   **d.** B. F. Skinner

FOR FURTHER CONSIDERATION

1. How can the health care professional prepare for working with various age groups?

2. Safety is an important issue for all age groups. How can you make your clinic safer for the various clients and visitors who frequent your facility?

3. How relevant is Freud's theory in today's health care setting?

4. Why is self-awareness such an important issue when working with the various age groups?

5. Now that you have finished this chapter, will there be any changes you will make personally in the way you communicate with various age groups? If so, identify the changes you will make and how you might implement them.

CASE STUDIES

Case Study 1

Catherine is 17½ years old. She has been seen by a pediatrician for childhood illnesses and checkups since she was born. Her mother and her grandmother both had thyroid cancer; since this a familial disorder, there is concern for Catherine. Her mother has annual follow-ups with an endocrinologist and has asked Catherine if she would allow him to check her blood and do an examination. This information could then be sent to the new internal medicine provider Catherine will be seeing as an adult.

1. How might her mother engage in conversation with Catherine? She does not want to cause undue concern or frighten Catherine.

2. Assuming Catherine agrees to visit the endocrinologist, how might he approach Catherine therapeutically?

3. What are some important considerations to think about when working with teenagers?

Case Study 2

Jim has a family history of coronary artery disease. His father had a massive heart attack and died at age 38. His twin brother had quadruple bypass surgery at age 42, and Jim had a mild heart attack at age 46. He has changed his lifestyle to reduce stress and include daily exercise; eats healthy, well-balanced meals; and monitors his cholesterol levels regularly. For the past 3 months, however, Jim has been experiencing atrial fibrillation and arrhythmia.

An important business meeting had Jim hurrying out the door with no time for breakfast and a 50-minute drive into the city through gridlock traffic. It was past lunchtime when he headed for home. While driving, he felt dizzy and pulled to the side of the freeway. He realized his heart was not functioning properly, but he had no chest pain or nausea. He called his cardiologist and was told to call 911 or get to the ER immediately. Jim, in denial, drove himself to the hospital, since he was only a few minutes away.

As Jim crossed the lobby of the ER, he experienced another dizzy spell and crashed into the counter. The receptionist asked him if that was his car in front of the door. He said, "Yes." The receptionist said, "You will have to move your car; you can't leave it there." Jim replied, "I'm having a heart attack, I need help!"

A passing nurse heard the comment and immediately went into action. Jim was soon on a gurney with six staff simultaneously poking and prodding his upper body.

An angiogram revealed that Jim had a 99% blockage in four of the main arteries of his heart, making quadruple bypass surgery a necessity. Jim is recovering nicely today and continues his healthy lifestyle.

1. How might the cardiologist have responded more therapeutically?

2. How would you classify the receptionist's response?

3. How might the receptionist have been more therapeutic?

REFERENCES AND RESOURCES

Frisch, N. C., & Frisch, L. E. (2010). *Psychiatric mental health nursing* (4th ed.). Clifton Park, NY: Delmar, Cengage Learning.

Mandleco, B. L. (2004). *Growth and development handbook: Newborn through adolescent*. Albany, NY: Thomson Delmar Learning.

Milliken, M. E., & Honeycutt, A. (2012). *Understanding human behavior: A guide for health care providers* (8th ed.). Clifton Park, NY: Delmar, Cengage Learning.

Pirkl, J. J. (n.d.). The demographics of aging. Retrieved from http://transgenerational.org/aging/demographics.htm.

United States Census Bureau. (2011). Census Bureau releases comprehensive analysis of fast-growing 90-and-older population. Retrieved from https://www.census.gov/newsroom/releases/archives/aging_population/cb11-194.html.

University of Cincinnati, Ohio. (2011). Aging and function: Examining impact on daily living. In *Look Closer, See Me* [Training modules]. Retrieved from www.nursing.uc.edu/content/dam/nursing/docs/CFAWD/LookCloserSeeMe/Module%202_GDST_Reference%20Guide.pdf.

Chapter 6

The Therapeutic Response to Stressed, Anxious, and Fearful Clients

CHAPTER OBJECTIVES

After completing this chapter, the learner should be able to:

- Define the key terms as presented in the glossary.
- Describe stress theories as presented by Claude Bernard, Walter B. Cannon, and Hans Selye.
- Differentiate between the terms stress and stressor(s).
- Diagram the stress response on the body.
- Describe the four stages of anxiety and appropriate therapeutic responses for each stage.
- Describe the behavior of a fearful client.
- Develop therapeutic approaches to a fearful client.
- List signs and symptoms of normal and dysfunctional stress in each age group.
- Describe ways to decrease stress for each age group.
- List the signs and symptoms of the client experiencing a panic attack.
- Provide a therapeutic response to the client experiencing a panic attack.
- Describe the stress-related disorders including social phobia, claustrophobia, necrophobia, blood-injury-injection phobia, obsessive–compulsive disorder, and posttraumatic stress disorder.

John and Janice live in a small community and completed a first-aid class several weeks ago. As Janice washed the lunch dishes one afternoon, she suddenly felt a sense of concern for the safety of her 5-year-old son, David, who was playing in the backyard. Hearing a scream, she ran to the window to see what had happened. Fear gripped Janice as she felt her heart pound and her stomach become tied in knots. From the window, she saw David lying on the ground, motionless. He had fallen from the treehouse where he often played.

When Janice reached David's side, she noticed how pale he was and that his voice was just a whimper. He felt cold and clammy, so she quickly removed her sweater and placed it gently around his limp body. Janice called to a neighbor to notify 911, and to bring some water and a washcloth. Janice comforted David and instructed him to lie still. When he asked for water, she gently touched his lips with the wet washcloth and then placed it on his forehead. David panted for air while Janice continued to speak softly to him and gently smoothed his hair back with her fingertips.

At the emergency room, x-rays revealed a broken leg, which was set and placed in a cast. David spent the night at the hospital for further observation and was discharged the next day.

Stop and Consider 6.1

Respond to the following questions:

1. What symptoms of stress and fear did Janice demonstrate in this scenario?

2. What symptoms of stress did David demonstrate?

3. How did Janice decrease stress for David while they waited for 911 to respond?

INTRODUCTION

The Chinese word for "crisis" is written by combining two symbols—one symbol meaning danger and the other meaning opportunity. **Stress** is just that: a danger and an opportunity, a friend and a foe.

Good stress, termed **eustress**, helps us cope with the challenges faced each day. Examples of good stress may include staying alert while driving to school or work, bringing tasks to mind that must be done, and assisting others during crisis. Eustress helps us feel energized, alert, in control, and able to make judgments and decisions.

Bad stress or **distress** is considered a danger or foe. When distress is experienced repeatedly or for a long duration, pathological changes may begin to occur. Examples of distress may include marriage preparations, divorce proceedings, raising a family, on-the-job difficulties, and the serious illness and/or death of a family member or close friend.

This chapter helps you recognize stressors, the effects of stress on health and well-being, and the possible consequences of long-duration stress. Stress management techniques and the impacts of stress through-out the life span are also discussed along with suggested therapeutic responses. Common stress-related disorders, such as panic attacks, phobias, obsessive–compulsive disorder, and posttraumatic stress disorder (PTSD) are discussed. Other stress-related disorders are discussed in Chapter 8. Learning to balance and manage stress leads to a healthier life.

STRESS THEORIES

Claude Bernard was a 19th-century French biologist who discovered that the body's internal milieu (internal environment) changed constantly to meet the daily demands of life. Blood pressure, heart rate, respiration, and the amount of available energy in the circulating blood supply fluctuate to maintain **homeostasis**. He also learned that if any of these changed too much, the body could not adapt, and death followed.

Sometimes outside agents, such as pathogens, injury and trauma, or environmental pollutants and contaminants, cause these changes to the body. Our bodies also have vulnerable spots. Disease and old injuries may leave weak areas that feel the impact of stress more quickly than other areas of the body. The aging process in general makes us more susceptible to stress symptoms.

Walter B. Cannon, a Harvard physiologist, went a step further than Bernard. Cannon discovered that the body adjusts when change threatens to be too great. For example, when a large amount of blood is lost through any means, the body compensates by causing small changes in blood vessels all over the body. The heart rate increases slightly and fluid is transferred from tissues to the bloodstream, to bring balance and homeostasis.

Cannon also discovered that when life-threatening situations arise, excitatory substances such as adrenaline, cortisol, and glucose are released into the bloodstream. These adjustments cause the body to adapt, and greatly enhance one's chances of survival. These substances prepare the body for effort and protect it from harm.

It was Hans Selye who first conceived the theory of nonspecific reactions to stress; he named his theory **general adaptation syndrome (GAS)**. Selye theorized that the body experiences four stages in its response to stress: (1) the alarm stage, (2) the fight-or-flight stage, (3) the exhaustion stage, and (4) the return-to-normal stage.

Selye also defined a resource he called *adaptive energy*. This energy influences the body's resistance to stress. It is inherited and varies from one individual to another. It consists of a superficial level that can be replenished at the conclusion of a stressful event and a deep level that is not replenished and, when depleted, results in disease or death.

The following paragraphs detail the four body responses Selye identified as part of GAS (Figure 6-1).

Alarm

The alarm stage is designed to sound a warning when something is perceived to create stress. Pain is a part of this system, as it tells us when body tissue is being damaged.

A therapeutic response in the medical setting would be to recognize the fact that pain does produce a stress response. When clients are in pain, blood pressure, pulse, and respiration rate may be elevated. Ask the client to describe the pain and how it feels. Where is the pain located? Is the pain constant or intermittent? Offer suggestions for coping with pain. Often,

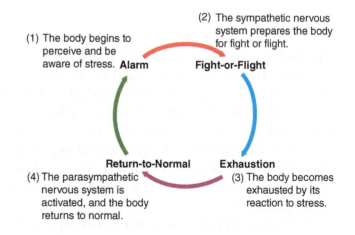

FIGURE 6-1   Hans Selye's general adaptation syndrome (GAS) theory proposes that four stages are involved in adapting to stress.

breathing in through the nose and exhaling through the mouth will help. If the pain is caused by a procedure in progress, you may be able to distract and engage the client in conversation, or reassure the client that it will soon be finished.

Fight or Flight

The **sympathetic nervous system** prepares the body for fight or flight. This response is particularly active when clients experience fear. The pupils dilate; the mouth becomes dry; and heart rate, pulse, and respiration all increase. Blood vessels in the skin constrict and blood vessels in the heart and brain dilate. There is decreased motility in the gastrointestinal and genitourinary tracts. All these changes prepare the body for whatever action may need to be taken.

 Health care professionals should be alert for these signs and take all possible measures to decrease the stress response. Recognize that a certain amount of stress will be present no matter why a client is seeing a provider. Clients may be concerned about how a procedure or illness will affect their physical, mental, and emotional well-being. They may be frustrated or angry because they do not have a solution to a particular problem. As a health care professional, it is important not to take anger that may be directed at you personally. It should be treated as a sign and symptom of a client's stress. Provide privacy for those who may be asked to disrobe for an examination. Knock on the door before entering. Keep equipment, instruments, and syringes covered or out of sight. It is very stressful to come into an examination room, see such items, and wonder how they will be used.

Professional

Exhaustion

The body can only stay in the fight-or-flight state for a limited time. Have you ever stretched a rubber band to the maximum and held it there? After a while, your body tires of holding the stretched rubber band and releases it. *When it is released, the band has lost some of its elasticity, which can never be recovered.* The same principle applies to the blood vessels throughout the body. After repeated periods of dilation and relaxation, they are weakened. *Also, if it is overstretched, the rubber band may snap.* Blood vessels burst when they are dilated to an extreme or have developed weakened areas.

Individuals in this stage of stress may experience physical fatigue. It is best not to give detailed instructions at this time. Rather, allow them time to recover—perhaps have them dress after the procedure and relax for a short while. If instructions must be given, it is best to write them out.

Return to Normal (Recovery)

During the return-to-normal stage, the **parasympathetic nervous system** kicks in and the body returns to normal. The pupils constrict; the salivary glands begin to function; and heart rate, pulse, and respiration decrease. Blood vessels dilate in the skin and constrict in the heart and brain. The gastrointestinal and genitourinary tracts begin to function again, and urinary urgency and/or diarrhea may be experienced.

In the medical setting, these individuals respond well to a calm, soft voice. Encourage them to talk about how they are feeling and what helps them cope with the stress. Eye contact and active listening skills will help as well.

STRESSORS AND STRESS

Life is full of hassles, inconveniences, frustrations, deadlines, and demands. A **stressor** is anything that causes stress. Stressors can come from internal or external sources and can be divided into four categories:

- *Frustrations:* These are circumstances that prevent us from doing what we want to do.
- *Conflicts:* Incompatibility between two important things or objectives equally important to us.
- *Pressure:* Demands of schedule, workload, or expectations placed on us by ourselves or others.
- *Fear:* Emotional reaction to immediate perceived danger resulting from real or imaginary situations or events.

Understanding the cause of stress is essential in order for stress management to be effective. The most common cause of stress is change; examples include relocation, job loss, job promotion, retirement, divorce, bereavement, illness, and the resultant fear from these changes.

The body does not differentiate between eustress and distress. It only considers the level of the stress and its duration. Stressors cause the body's **autonomic nervous system** to respond, to protect the body. This places the body in a state of stress that can be beneficial or harmful, depending on severity and duration.

Internal stressors are products of emotions and result in anxiety. Internal stressors can be totally imaginary, having no relationship to real events. Persistent thoughts that reflect exaggerated fear produce internal stressors that can lead to obsessive–compulsive disorder. An example might be the fear of germs. A client may be constantly washing his or her hands or be afraid to touch anything that is perceived as contaminated. Memories or nonthreatening real events can also trigger internal stressors as representative of military personnel returning from combat and upon hearing a car backfire experience flashbacks of their war experiences.

External stressors result from external events or observations and involve a sensation of fright or fearfulness. The body's response is the same as for internal stressors, except that the duration of the stress is controlled by the external event. Most external stressors are of short duration. An example of a short-term external stressor would be a dog suddenly lunging toward you. An example of a longer-duration external stressor would be a soldier in continuous combat lasting days, weeks, or months. Initially the fear factor is very high, resulting in many soldiers feeling emotionally numb or causing them to disassociate themselves. With time, the external stressor becomes the norm but can lead to PTSD after combat ends. Stressors that are severe or have a long duration may become medically significant forms of mental illness. Various forms of depression can also result from stress. These are discussed fully in Chapter 8.

ANXIETY

Internal stressors are created in the mind and are sometimes classified as "emotional allergies." **Anxiety** is the normal response to this type of stressor. It is a feeling of apprehension, worry, uneasiness, or dread frequently accompanied by physical symptoms, much as in the fight-or-flight stage. Anxiety is different from fear. Fear is the reaction to a known and usually an external threat. Anxiety, on the other hand, may occur at any time, develops from within, and may be triggered by any situation. The level of anxiety is the key issue. There are four levels of anxiety: mild, moderate, severe, and panic.

Mild Anxiety

Mild anxiety is routinely experienced in normal everyday living. It is considered healthy, as it increases perception. During mild anxiety, our body functions well. It is stimulated by the increased production of adrenaline and cortisol, which enables us to think clearly and focus on details; to be alert, organized, and efficient; and to make wise decisions and judgments. While experiencing mild anxiety, memory retention and learning are heightened.

Therapeutic responses to the person experiencing mild anxiety include providing details for health care and instructions and offering choices regarding treatment when decisions must be made.

Moderate Anxiety

The person experiencing moderate anxiety has decreased perception. Their focus is on a particular task or problem rather than on the overall circumstance. When experiencing moderate anxiety, the individual will still be alert and able to think clearly. Concentration, however, will be focused on one challenge at a time. Decisions and judgments will be made on each individual detail as it is experienced or as the person becomes aware of another detail.

An example of moderate anxiety could be a driver passing through a school zone with a speed camera. The driver tends to focus totally on the speedometer, ignoring students in a crosswalk. This could create a very dangerous situation.

Therapeutic responses include focusing on one detail at a time; speaking in a soft, calm manner; encouraging relaxed breathing techniques; and keeping the person informed regarding how much longer the procedure will take or the time when the discomfort will be over. Sometimes just saying "You seem very anxious today" will help the person let go of some of the stress.

Severe Anxiety

During severe anxiety, individuals experience an inability to focus on details, or they may be able to focus attention only on one aspect of a situation. Abstract thinking is lost. Some concrete directions may be followed, but learning generally does not take place. Because of the inability to concentrate, these individuals will be very indecisive.

Therapeutic responses to severe anxiety include giving detailed instructions to a family member or writing out the instructions for the client. Give clients brochures or pamphlets to read after they have had time to gain self-control. Telephone later in the day or the next day to see how they are doing or if they have any questions.

Panic Anxiety

Panic anxiety can occur with little or no warning and most often is a response to some stressor. The individual may experience a racing heart rate or shortness of breath and may feel they have some life-threatening

TABLE 6-1   **Signs and Symptoms for the Four Levels of Anxiety**

Mild anxiety	Minor muscle tension, normal behavior, relaxed, normal vital signs, broad focus, alert
Moderate anxiety	Moderately tense, very attentive, energetic, enhanced level of concern, slightly elevated vital signs, focused on stressor
Severe anxiety	Tense, increased pulse and blood pressure with shallow breathing, tunnel vision, short temper, lack of appetite or binge eating or drinking, limited problem-solving ability, short attention span, shaky or high-pitched voice
Panic	Loss of emotional control, irrational, show symptoms related to shock, gasping for breath, possible chest pain, mental depression, loss of problem-solving capability, disorganized

illness. These symptoms are generally short-lived and once the stressor is gone the anxiety and symptoms disappear. During the panic anxiety stage, individuals are consumed with escape. They want to remove themselves from the situation. Communication may be difficult, rational thinking and concentration is diminished, and the person becomes increasingly active without any directed purpose. Pacing and jumping from task to task are common characteristics of a person experiencing panic anxiety. Panic anxiety can be hereditary or the result of life experiences.

Therapeutic approaches for panic anxiety are the same as for severe anxiety. It is important not to allow a person in this state to leave the clinic until recovery has taken place or until someone else can drive the person home. Table 6-1 provides a summary of the signs and symptoms for the four levels of anxiety. A review of Maslow's Hierarchy of Needs found in Appendix A is helpful in assessing the needs of those experiencing various levels of anxiety.

THE FEARFUL CLIENT

Fear is an emotion aroused primarily by something you are uncertain of or by some sort of threat, whether real or imagined. There are different degrees of fear, and fear varies with each individual. Fear can lead to social problems if not appropriately addressed. Fear has many definitions, but some are distrust, worry, dread, fright, paranoia, or terror.

Case Study: Fearful Client

Harry, a 49-year-old construction worker recuperating from a myocardial infarction, returns to the medical clinic for a follow-up evaluation. Harry is uncooperative; Dr. Cooper discovers that Harry is not taking his anticoagulants, is back to work a month prior to the recommended time, and is still chain-smoking. Harry is quite agitated and secretly believes that if he ignores his heart issue, it will all go away. Today he fears that Dr. Cooper will be quite unhappy with his noncompliance and is not sure he can face the consequences he knows for certain he will hear about.

Stop and Consider 6.2

1. Is Harry using any defense mechanism and, if so, which one(s)?

2. If you were Dr. Cooper, what would your therapeutic response be to Harry?

Distrust and worry are emotions that usually focus on a person or object. The fear is gone when the person or object disappears. For example, when a client is fearful of a blood draw, distrust of the laboratory technician and worry about the discomfort can induce fear. Once the blood is drawn, the band aid in place, and the client leaves the area, the fear subsides.

Dread is the fear usually experienced prior to an event. A client who shrinks back when a nurse approaches the hospital bed with a syringe in hand knows what is coming and dreads the event. Harry displays a great deal of dread in the Case Study.

Paranoia is a psychosis of fear that is related to a feeling of being victimized. Paranoia can cause irrational or compulsive behavior. Women who have been unsuccessful in getting pregnant and who are desperate to give birth to a child may break down in uncontrollable sobs when they discover that another menstrual period has begun. They wonder why this happens to them.

A hospital housekeeper who simply cannot get her cleaning supplies from the closet because she sees a spider web with a large ugly spider is exhibiting terror. *Terror* occurs when an individual is overwhelmed with a feeling of impending danger. This kind of fear may cause an illogical reaction and is a form of panic attack. **Suppression** of fear may eventually turn into *somatic* symptoms. (Refer to Appendix B.)

A client's **denial** of fear may be an unconscious *defense mechanism*—an attempt to protect oneself by blocking an emotionally painful experience. People using this mechanism are unable to recognize the cause of their discomfort and may even deny being frightened or fearful. Some clients can be so threatened by their illnesses that they will not permit themselves to be aware of their feelings. These clients tend to be hypercritical of treatment and unusually demanding. It is difficult for these clients to accept help from their caregivers, since to do so is to acknowledge their fears.

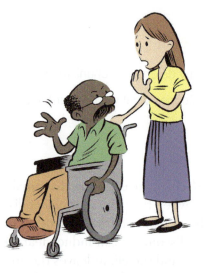

"BUZZ OFF. I CAN DO IT."

The Therapeutic Response

It is important to recognize and accept the client's fears. Statements such as "This can be very frightening" help a client feel accepted even though fear has been exhibited.

The problem-solving approach often reveals an acceptable solution. Once the client visualizes a solution, the fear begins to decrease.

Allow the client as much control over the situation as possible. When clients feel in control of the treatment, they are less fearful. Explain procedures and treatments carefully, taking time to assure clients and allay their fears. A client can feel fear even if he or she has an extensive medical background.

Act for the client who is panic-stricken. Such people are unable to act for themselves and need the assistance of others. For instance, a person listening to her best friend's panic over a lump in her breast may pick up the phone to make an appointment with a provider for her friend, and also go with her to the appointment. When panic occurs in the health care setting, stay with the client until the panic subsides. If appropriate, explain the situation to the partner or friend who may accompany the client. With the hospital housekeeper in a panic over the spider, another employer can be called to be with her, assure her that the spider is more fearful of her than vice versa, offer to get supplies for her, and also get rid of the spider and the web.

STRESS AND THE LIFE SPAN

It is interesting to note that all age groups from infant to older adult experience stress in varying degrees throughout each day. All cultures and genders experience stress as well, though they may respond to the stress in different ways. Men and women, for example, respond differently to stress. Men often become physically or verbally aggressive, and may also use denial as a defense mechanism. (See Appendix B for more information on defense mechanisms.) Women, on the other hand, often internalize their stress, mulling it over and over again in their minds. This reaction may lead to depression if satisfactory solutions to the stress are not achieved. The following paragraphs describe the possible impacts of stress throughout the life span and offer therapeutic responses and suggestions for ways to decrease stress.

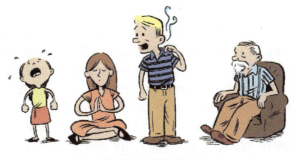

"EVERYBODY DEALS WITH
STRESS DIFFERENTLY."

Infants and Toddlers

Early experiences greatly influence behavior patterns in later life. It is not so much what happens during infancy, but what does *not* happen that has an impact on behavioral patterns. An infant is totally dependent upon adults for survival. For the infant, the method of expressing stress is to cry. While you may not always be able to shield the infant from stressful events, your relationship with the infant will serve as a buffer to stressful situations.

When parents fail to show interest in the infant, and the infant's needs are not satisfied, certain behavioral patterns are recognizable at the toddler stage. Often the toddler will display a lack of interest in others and experience limited or below-average communication skills. They may even revert to a more infantile stage that helps them feel more loved and secure.

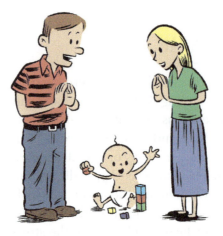

"GOOD JOB, DANNY. THAT'S
A NICE TOWER."

The Therapeutic Response

To reduce stress, the infant's physical and emotional needs must be met. Health care professionals must recognize the fact that not all parents understand or have the basic skills and financial resources to meet these needs. Provide community resource materials to parents and caregivers and take time to teach and instruct when appropriate. Be aware of safety issues within the facility and take measures to correct any hazards. At each visit carefully observe infants and toddlers for any signs that might indicate abuse or neglect and follow clinic protocols for reporting any such findings. Hold infants and speak soothingly to them, especially after any painful procedure. Nurturing behaviors such as smiling, rubbing the infant's back, or gently patting their bottom are comforting and help reduce stress.

Therapeutic responses for toddlers include consistency. As much as possible keep clinic visits routine. Speak directly to toddlers at their eye level and be honest with them. If they ask if it will hurt, describe how it might feel—like a bee sting or like a pinch. Praising toddlers for their accomplishments, no matter how small the feat, will build self-confidence and encourage a willingness to keep trying new things. If appropriate, discuss good parenting skills including nutrition and proper sleep for toddlers to boost their coping skills.

School-Age Children

School-age children experience a great deal of stress as they begin the transitional activities between home and school. Suddenly the security of everything known to the child is shaken. Children may express stress based on their stage of growth and development, or may reflect patterns of dealing with stress demonstrated by other family members or caregivers. Children generally exhibit fear easier than adults before they become so conditioned by the words, "There is nothing to be afraid of." When children feel threatened, they may revert to a more infantile behavior; this is termed **regression**. (See Appendix B.) Examples of such behavior include bed-wetting, hair-twirling, thumb sucking, or stuttering. Other signals of stress during this time period are nail-biting, a decreased appetite, headaches, and stomachaches.

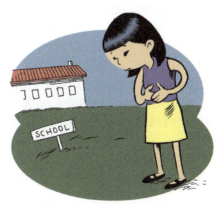

"OH, MY TUMMY HURTS."

The Therapeutic Response

Provide community resources and educational materials to parents and caregivers, taking time to teach and instruct when appropriate. Discuss proper rest and good nutrition with parents and caregivers as a means of boosting coping skills. Explain each procedure using terms the child will understand. Be honest with children and take time to answer their questions and concerns. Give children choices when possible and provide encouragement and praise for accomplishments. If children demonstrate their stress through acting-out behavior that expresses their frustrations (e.g., throwing things), do not respond in an authoritarian manner, rather provide stress reducing alternatives. Offer the child a pillow to punch or materials to draw a picture that expresses their feelings.

Adolescents

Case Study: Adolescent Stress

Ariana is almost 17 years old and has not seen her pediatrician for a few years. She needs to schedule her first pelvic exam. Ariana has a history of blood-injury-injection phobia, sometimes referred to as "white coat syndrome." When she was much younger, she fainted at her first dentist appointment, and has fainted when seeing the pediatrician for the first time. Ariana has also fainted at the chiropractic clinic and when she went with her boyfriend to get his tattoo. Because of her age, the same pediatrician explains that she needs to transition to a primary care provider (PCP) for her adult care and refers Ariana to one in the same building. She offers to transfer her medical records to the new PCP.

The appointment has been scheduled and now that the day has arrived Ariana is very anxious. This will be her first pelvic examination. Ariana hopes this provider has seen her medical history. The medical assistant (MA) asks the reason for her visit and Ariana feels her entire body tighten and she gets warm all over. Her vital signs are taken and the MA explains that the provider will be in shortly.

Ariana sits in a chair waiting and becoming more and more anxious and fearful. When the provider enters she tells her that her blood pressure is a little *high and asks if she has a history of hypertension. Ariana isn't sure what that means so she just looks at the provider. They begin to talk about the reason for the visit, but Ariana faints and falls off the chair, striking her head on the edge of the exam table. Since the new provider has not looked at Ariana's medical record carefully she does not understand Ariana's white coat syndrome and thinks she has had a seizure and 911 is called, further stressing and embarrassing Ariana. The medics take her to the ER where, again, she is further traumatized. Her mother has been called and upon arrival tries to piece what happened together. After bloodwork comes back from the lab, Ariana is diagnosed with nothing more than fainting and is discharged.*

Stop and Consider 6.3

1. How might the new PCP have reduced stress for a new client upon entering the examination room? What, if anything, might Ariana have done when she arrived at the clinic for her appointment?

2. What physical signs of stress did Ariana exhibit that would alert the provider she was stressed?

Adolescence is defined as a period of change. The body is in the process of changing from a child to an adult. The development of breasts, narrowing of the waist and widening of the hips, growth of axillary and pubic hair, hormonal changes, and menstruation are some changes females experience. Males begin to broaden through the shoulders and develop upper-body strength; facial, axillary, and pubic hair grows. They may experience acne, hormonal changes, and a cracking voice. Growth spurts may make them awkward and clumsy.

Adolescents experience social demands and peer pressure as well. They are still children, yet in many ways are considered men or women. They are expected to make decisions regarding college and career goals, and they often begin their search for a mate. Adolescents begin to explore their sexuality. Peer pressure is a huge factor in their lives, and they begin to think about emancipation from family. Becoming more autonomous and independent are key focuses.

The Therapeutic Response

Therapeutic responses to adolescents may include providing educational and community resource material as well as taking time to teach and instruct when appropriate. Provide for their privacy needs and respect their modesty. Allow plenty of time to disrobe and show them where to put clothing items. Knock before entering the room. Explain procedures in terms they will understand and respond to all of their questions. Give adolescents choices when possible.

Adults

Adults experience a variety of stressors. Mortgage payments, career commitments, and perhaps marriage and a family are just a few. Often adults are overloaded with too much to do and not enough time to do it. Many adults find themselves experiencing the "sandwich syndrome." Today's trend is to begin a family later in life, with many adults becoming first-time parents at the age of 35 or 40. This means their children are still under their roof when they begin to have responsibility for aging parents. They are caught in the middle, or sandwiched, between the two generations. Teenagers and aging parents both require intense energy expenditures and create many stressors.

Some parents may experience the "boomerang generation." Children who have been out of the home 4 or 5 years are now graduating from college, may have huge college debts to repay, and are not able to financially support themselves. They "boomerang" back home to live with their parents until they earn and save enough money to afford to move out on their own.

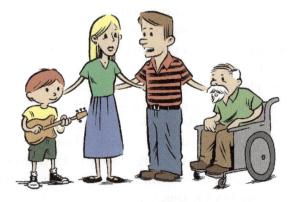

THE SANDWICH GENERATION
FAMILY

The Therapeutic Response

Adults cope with stress better when they have a network of friends and/or colleagues with whom they can share. It is always helpful to know that others are experiencing similar feelings, and to learn how they are coping with them. Additional therapeutic responses to the adult may include providing educational and resource material as appropriate. Answer all of their questions completely and encourage verbalization regarding their feelings. Discuss treatment plans and provide options when possible. The benefits of a healthy lifestyle including nutrition, exercise, sleep, and avoiding alcohol and recreational drugs may be discussed as a means of decreasing stress.

Older Adults

Case Study: Older Adult Stress

Mrs. Rodriguez has been told by her optometrist that she needs to see an ophthalmologist to discuss cataract surgery. Mrs. Rodriguez is 80 years old and has been living in an assisted-living environment for the past 4 years. She seems alert and is trying to listen carefully to the instructions but does not comprehend all of them and is becoming frustrated. Dr. Jones asks if Mrs. Rodriguez has a family member who can drive her on the day of surgery and take her home. He also asks if someone will be with her for the first 24 hours after surgery and who can also drive her to a follow-up appointment the day after surgery. Dr. Jones provides printed information explaining the procedure and what to expect after the surgery.

Stop and Consider 6.4

1. How might Mrs. Rodriguez's stress differ from a younger adult?

2. Identify important therapeutic considerations when dealing with older adults.

Older adults face many stressors; among these are retirement, illness, and death. Much of an older person's stress comes from loss rather than gain. They are slowing down physically and mentally. The body deteriorates and wears out. The mind is not as alert and it is difficult to remember things that were once so important. There is a loss of energy, agility, beauty, and family togetherness. Retirement brings the loss of a job, perhaps other losses of security, finances, structure, routine, independence, and relationships.

The Therapeutic Response

Older adults have raised their family and employment stress is a thing of the past, but the challenge of declining health, financial concerns, and isolation take their place. Therapeutic responses to older adults may include providing educational and resource materials. Taking time to answer all of their questions and concerns is critical. Show older adults respect by addressing them by their full name and title and do not use endearing terms such as "dear," "sweetie," or "honey." Ask for their opinion when appropriate and allow them to make decisions regarding their health care when possible. Encourage emotional support such as involvement in community centers and exercise programs such as Medicare's Silver Sneakers program.

STRESS-RELATED DISORDERS

A few stress-related disorders are discussed in the following paragraphs. Various types of depression, also related to stress, are discussed in Chapter 8.

Severe anxiety, fear, and panic are terrifying for the individual experiencing them, and may manifest themselves in more serious stress-related disorders. It is sometimes difficult to differentiate between severe anxiety and panic attacks. Panic attacks, however, are unprovoked and unpredictable, but also may be the result of an external stressor. Panic attacks may last up to an hour and often leave a client feeling exhausted. These fears are abnormal when they interfere with daily living activities or when they cause an individual to take extreme measures to avoid the feared experience. Extreme measures of avoidance may lead to various types of phobias.

Intense fear, sometimes known as phobia, impacts the lives of some individuals daily. Not much is known about the cause of phobias; however, there may be some connection between phobias children have and the phobias their parents have. The most common phobias likely witnessed by health care professionals include social phobia, claustrophobia, necrophobia, and blood-injury-injection phobia.

Professionalism

As a health care professional if you experience any of these phobias yourself or are uncomfortable with clients experiencing these disorders, you may find more satisfying work as an administrative assistant as opposed to one giving direct medical attention.

Obsessive–compulsive disorder is an obsession with irrational upsetting thoughts that cause anxiety and fear in the person with no seeming external stressor. Women are twice as susceptible to this disorder as men. Clients suffering from this disorder use rituals such as nail-biting, hair-pulling, or handwashing to attempt to control the anxiety and fear their thoughts produce. It may be nearly impossible for these clients to communicate with the health care professional because they are so focused on the need to perform the ritual.

Posttraumatic stress syndrome (PTSD) results from reliving a traumatic event through conscious thoughts or in the form of nightmares during sleep. It can be triggered by ordinary events or by events having similarity to the actual traumatic occurrence. The person experiencing PTSD may lose touch with reality during the event. PTSD can lead to depression, substance abuse, and other anxiety disorders if left untreated.

SUMMARY

Stress is part of life, no matter what age group a client represents. Stressors signal the body to go into alarm, and may be caused by anything—fear, worry, threat, or even challenging events. Eustress helps the body function efficiently, make judgments and decisions, and work at peak performance. Distress may be harmful to the body and is related to the intensity and duration of the stressor.

Anxiety is a feeling of apprehension, worry, uneasiness, or dread frequently accompanied by physical symptoms, much as in the fight-or-flight stage of stress. Anxiety develops from within and may arise in response to perceived or real events. A client's denial of fear may be an unconscious defense mechanism. Stress, anxiety, and fear that is not managed may lead to the development of more serious diseases and disorders.

Health care professionals who understand human growth and development issues will be able to recognize stressors in their clients no matter what their age. Age-appropriate therapeutic responses will encourage clients to verbalize their feelings and concerns. Being able to suggest ways to manage or reduce stress is also helpful for clients.

EXERCISES

Exercise 1

Determining how well you handle stress will help identify personal strengths and weaknesses and point you toward the skills needed to be a successful health care professional. Complete the following stress self-test.

How Stressed Are You????

Score each statement as a 0, 1, 2, 3, or 4.

0 = never; 1 = rarely; 2 = sometimes; 3 = often; 4 = very often/always

Instructions for scoring follow the statements.

_____	1) My sleep is poor—delayed onset, wake early, or not restful
_____	2) I have headaches regularly (tension or migraine)
_____	3) I feel tense and anxious
_____	4) I rarely have enough time to complete tasks
_____	5) I experience frustration when trying to get things accomplished
_____	6) I feel like escaping; I wish I were somewhere else
_____	7) I feel like my schedule is controlled by outside factors or other people
_____	8) I feel angry even for no reason
_____	9) I feel overwhelmed by things that shouldn't be that hard
_____	10) I eat more sugar and junk food than I want
_____	11) I am not happy with the way I look
_____	12) I have digestive difficulties (gas, cramping, irregularity)
_____	13) I feel like I want to cry; I am tearful more often than normal
_____	14) I can't concentrate
_____	15) I have constant colds/flu/infections
_____	16) I feel isolated even when around others
_____	17) I am forgetful; even important things slip my mind
_____	18) I have pain in more than one place in my body
_____	19) I feel irritable
_____	20) I am unorganized and lose things
_____	21) I have cold hands and or feet
_____	22) I am late for appointments or meetings
_____	23) I have moist or sweaty hands
_____	24) I talk rapidly
_____	25) My heart pounds in my chest

Scoring

Add all your points together. You can have a total of 100 points. The higher the score, the greater your stress response. Keep in mind that your symptoms may not be just stress related—it is important to see your provider if you are not feeling well!

0–25—low

26–36—low-moderate

37–50—moderate-high

50–65—high

+65—very high

© John Jordy, The Stress Clinic, LLC

Exercise 2

Briefly describe your therapeutic response to the following situations. These exercises can be used in small group settings or can be completed independent of others.

1. Your client presents at the dentist's clinic experiencing moderate anxiety and is consumed with only that particular problem. Your therapeutic response includes _____

   _____

   _____

2. A new mom brings her infant to the pediatrician for his 6-week checkup. Both appear very stressed. Your therapeutic response to the mom includes _____

   _____

   _____

   Your therapeutic response to the infant includes _____

   _____

   _____

3. Fourteen-year-old Kenji arrives for his scheduled appointment. He appears very shy and nervous, and finally tells you he came because of his acne. Your therapeutic response includes _____

   _____

   _____

4. Your client and his wife arrive at the ambulatory care clinic because Alex thinks he is having a heart attack. After seeing the provider, he is diagnosed with panic anxiety.
Your therapeutic response includes _____

_____

_____

5. Rachael is very upset because the school nurse told her daughter Ty that she had scoliosis. Rachael made an appointment with the chiropractor for a complete examination, including x-rays.
Your therapeutic response to Rachael includes _____

_____

_____

Your therapeutic response to Ty includes _____

_____

_____

Exercise 3

Using the Internet, look for self-help, bulletin boards, or other electronic reference sources that could help you, family members, or clients understand and manage stress. Make a list of the resources you have found to be shared with the class.

Exercise 4

Using Appendix A, review the age groups as discussed by each theorist. Identify potential stressors for each age group. Now, write a therapeutic response for each stressor listed.

REVIEW QUESTIONS

Multiple Choice

1. Hans Selye's general adaptation syndrome theory proposes that adaptation to stress occurs in how many stages?
   a. Two stages   c. Four stages
   b. Three stages   d. Five stages

2. Which statement best describes mild anxiety?

   a. May include physiological changes such as perspiration and increased heart and respiratory rates

   b. May include behavioral manifestations such as irritability and pacing

   c. May include inability to focus on details or focusing on only one aspect of a situation

   d. Is considered healthy because it enables one to think clearly, focus on details, and to make wise decisions and judgments

3. During panic anxiety, therapeutic responses include which of the following?

   a. Providing details and instructions for health care that are appropriate.

   b. Giving detailed instructions to a family member or in writing to the client.

   c. Focusing on one detail at a time, keeping the client informed.

   d. Offering choices regarding treatment decisions.

4. Which response is not a way to decrease stress?

   a. Aerobic activity   **c.** Mediation

   b. Planning ahead and   **d.** Enjoying caffeine or alcohol often
   being organized

5. The sympathetic nervous system prepares the body for which phase of the GAS theory?

   a. Exhaustion   **c.** Alarm

   b. Fight or flight   **d.** Return to normal

6. What is the term for internal perceptions or external events that cause the body to protect itself?

   a. Stressors   **c.** Sympathetic nervous system

   b. Stress   **d.** Parasympathetic nervous system

7. Which method does an infant use to express stress?

   a. Throwing things   **c.** Crying

   b. Regression   **d.** Hair-twirling

8. Which therapeutic response is appropriate for adolescents?

   a. Hold them and speak soothingly

   b. Discuss treatment plans and provide options

   c. Allow them to make decisions about their health care

   d. Allow for privacy and respect their modesty

9. Which type of anxiety is described in the following statement? Communication may be difficult, rational thinking and concentration is diminished, pacing and jumping from task to task.

   a. Panic anxiety   **c.** Severe anxiety

   b. Mild anxiety   **d.** Moderate anxiety

10. What is the meaning of eustress?

   a. Bad stress   **c.** Panic anxiety

   b. Anxiety   **d.** Good stress

FOR FURTHER CONSIDERATION

1. How can health care professionals help the caregiver living with chronic stress while caring for an older parent with Alzheimer's around the clock?

2. How do men and women respond differently to stress? Give specific examples.

3. How does understanding human growth and development aid the health care professional to assess and deal with stress and the life cycle?

CASE STUDIES

Case Study 1

Elizabeth, a 68-year-old woman, has experienced relatively good health for most of her lifetime. A year and a half ago, she suffered a bout of pneumonia, with a very difficult recovery. She continued to "feel sick," and had no appetite. Weight loss and decreased energy levels ensued. Her primary care provider admitted her to the hospital for further tests, which revealed a diagnosis of chronic obstructive pulmonary disease (COPD) (although she had never been a smoker), and pulmonary aspergillosis. She was discharged with a PICC (peripherally inserted central catheter) line and daily administration of antibiotics at the IV therapy center. After 3 months of IV therapy, the aspergillosis seemed to be gone and Elizabeth felt somewhat healthier.

Houseguests visited Elizabeth during the summer, and one of them came down with a cold. With permanent damage from the COPD, a weakened immune system, and the trauma and stress that Elizabeth had just been through, she caught the cold, which developed into another bout of pneumonia. The aspergillosis returned and a pulmonary embolism and blood clot were found in her left leg. The PICC line was reinserted and Coumadin prescribed. This treatment meant daily trips to the IV therapy center and a stop at the hospital lab to have Coumadin levels evaluated.

1. What indicators of stress do you see manifested in this case study?

2. How can Elizabeth better deal with this stress?

3. How can health care professionals help her manage the stress?

Case Study 2

Juan is 3½ years old when a new sister joins the family. At first Juan is excited about having a new sister, because family members bring him presents and he also gets to open gifts brought for his sister. But when she cries, Mom is prompt to attend to her needs and Juan has to wait until his sister is settled before Mom can help him. Juan thinks it takes a long time for his sister to get her bath and eat her meals. He becomes frustrated at not receiving all of Mom's attention and begins to act out by shouting and sometimes throwing toys. Juan, who has been toilet trained for some time, begins to soil his pants and wants to drink from a sippy cup again, rather than using his grown-up plastic cup.

1. What steps can his mother take to decrease Juan's stress and frustration?

2. According to Erikson, which stage of development is Juan experiencing? (See Appendix A.)

3. What defense mechanism is Juan demonstrating? (See Appendix B.)

REFERENCES AND RESOURCES

American Psychiatric Association (2013). *Diagnostic and statistical manual of mental disorders* (5th ed.). Arlington, VA: Author.

Frisch, N. C., & Frisch, L. E. (2010). *Psychiatric mental health nursing* (4th ed.). Clifton Park, NY: Cengage Learning.

Lindh, W. Q., Pooler, M. S., Tamparo, C. D., & Dahl, B. M. (2014). *Comprehensive medal assisting: Administrative and clinical competencies* (5th ed.). Clifton Park, NY: Cengage Learning.

Mandleco, B. L. (2004). *Growth and development handbook: Newborn through adolescent*. Albany, NY: Thomson Delmar Learning.

Milliken, M. E. (2012). *Understanding human behavior* (8th ed.). Clifton Park, NY: Cengage Learning.

National Institute of Mental Health. (2015, May). Anxiety disorders. Retrieved March 3, 2015, from www.nimh.nih.gov/health/publications/anxiety-disorders/index.shtml?rf=53414.

Tamparo, C. D. (2016). *Diseases of the human body* (6th ed.). Philadelphia: F. A. Davis.

Chapter 7

The Therapeutic Response to Angry, Aggressive, Abused, or Abusive Clients

CHAPTER OBJECTIVES

After completing this chapter, the learner should be able to:

- Define key terms as presented in the glossary.

- Differentiate the angry from the aggressive client.

- List at least four descriptors of inappropriate aggressive behavior.

- Identify at least five therapeutic approaches to the angry or aggressive client.

- Summarize likely characteristics of an abuser.

- Discuss the three phases of violence.

- Describe four types of abuse.

- Identify what constitutes intimate partner violence (IPV), child abuse and neglect, and older adult abuse and neglect.

- Contrast the three categories used to identify rapists.

- Explain the crisis stages experienced by rape survivors.

- Recall treatment protocol for abused individuals.

- Explain documentation and reporting guidelines for instances of abuse.

- Discuss therapeutic responses to both the abuser and the abused.

- Examine personal attitudes toward anger, aggression, and abuse.

Opening Case Study

A 36-year-old woman dressed in a power suit and carrying a briefcase hurriedly approaches the pharmacy counter in a large national-chain drug store. The professional behind the counter (a pharmacy assistant) is caring for a customer at the drive-up window.

Customer: (clears her throat loudly) "Excuse me, but I need a prescription filled, and I am in a hurry."

Pharmacy Assistant: "I'm almost finished here. The pharmacist has stepped out for just a moment; he will assist you as soon as he returns."

Customer: "What do you mean, the pharmacist isn't here? Can't you help me?"

The pharmacy assistant, now finished with the drive-up window customer, looks at the prescription and says, "We can have this filled for you in 15 minutes."

Customer: (now clearly agitated) "Fifteen minutes! I haven't got all day. I came here, to this discount drug store, because I thought you would be faster than my regular pharmacist. I had to wait 45 minutes on the doctor, and now I have to wait on you. I will never make my afternoon appointment. Just throw those damn pills in a bottle and tell me what it costs."

Pharmacy Assistant: "Sorry, I can't do that."

Customer: "Then give me back my prescription; I'll go someplace where I can get some service."

Pharmacy Assistant: (tosses the prescription back at the customer) "Good riddance."

The pharmacist returns just as the customer storms away and says to him, "Fire that incompetent witch."

Stop and Consider 7.1

1. Identify the stressors the customer exhibited.

2. When did the stress become anger?

3. What happened to cause the pharmacy assistant to respond as she did?

4. What might be a therapeutic response in this situation?

INTRODUCTION

Professionalism

🎗 The therapeutic response implies that the health care professional will be relating to people in need. Often these people will be frustrated, angry, and even aggressive. Sometimes they are abusive or abused. Recognizing and understanding such behavior enables the professional to more easily respond in a therapeutic manner.

THE ANGRY CLIENT

Case Study: An Angry Client

James approaches your desk to make another appointment. He is obviously agitated. He slaps a piece of paper on the counter. You recognize it as a diet the provider has prescribed for his diabetic condition. He sarcastically says to you, "It is impossible to stay on this diet! Who does that doctor think she is?"

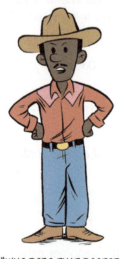

"WHO DOES THAT DOCTOR
THINK SHE IS?"

Anger is an emotion that may be brought on by frustration, threats, obstacles, or offensive situations. In most cases anger is temporary, and is often directed toward a specific object or person. *Annoyance* is a term used to describe a mild form of anger, and *resentment* is a chronic form of anger that is long lasting. Intense anger or animosity directed toward a particular person or people is termed *hatred*. Any form of anger that is not resolved may have a negative impact on one's behavior after an extended period.

Inappropriate expression of anger includes hostility that is displaced or physically acted out against another person. Such anger can lead to injury or harm to another person. (See **displacement** in Appendix B.) Hostility is displaced when it is directed toward someone or something other than the cause of the frustration. If a person is angry over circumstances at work but takes it out on the family cat when returning home, this is displaced hostility. Anger that is not properly managed easily turns into aggression.

Every human being experiences anger. What is done with anger is the key to a healthy mental attitude. Anger can generate positive energy. If the emotion encourages an individual to find a solution to a problem, changes an unhealthy lifestyle, or manifests itself in appropriate physical activity, the anger is not turned inward to breed contempt or cause physical ailments later.

Clients who are angry are often easy to recognize. They have an angry tone in their voice and in their facial expression; they may use profanity. Generally, they talk rapidly and rarely listen. Angry clients usually feel frustrated and annoyed. The frustration can come from any number of sources and may or may not be correctly addressed to the health care professional. James's frustration, in the previous case study, may be over a diet he cannot follow because (1) he likes little or none of the foods, (2) he is afraid he cannot follow the diet, (3) he is afraid he's losing control over his life, or (4) he is dealing with some totally unrelated incident in his life.

Health care professionals will, from time to time, experience angry comments made by clients. To understand and cope with these comments, some recommendations follow.

The Therapeutic Response

Professionalism

- *Do not take offense at a client's comments or take them personally.* Evaluate the actions on their merit, not as a personal affront. This requires control, patience, and a healthy self-esteem on the part of the health care professional.

- *A demanding client may really be lonely, anxious, frightened, or insecure.* Give reassurance and offer explanations of services or procedures. Try to determine what the client really needs to be comfortable and work toward a solution.

- *Accept clients as they are.* Help your clients regain their self-esteem by talking out their angry feelings. "You seem quite upset about this

(continues)

The Therapeutic Response   (*Continued*)

new diet" is a comment that encourages James to tell more about his hostile feelings, but does not make him feel ashamed.

- *Use techniques to de-escalate client anger.* Speak in a calm, reassuring voice and at a slightly slower pace than usual. Use controlled expressions. Let the client know that anger is an appropriate emotion, but gently indicate what you will not be able to accept.

- *Be patient and do not rush interactions.* Allow clients to express their anger in a controlled, unhurried atmosphere. Often, just being able to verbalize frustrations calms an individual who is angry. Once the client is calm, return to a solution to the problem without further mention of the anger.

- *Listen carefully to verbal and nonverbal communication.* Remember the communication cycle. The message may have to be decoded and checked for its validity to determine the real message. Health care professionals may find it difficult to listen because they are anxious to defend their position.

- *Do not defend or blame.* Do as much as possible to help resolve the problem. Do not argue with the client; to do so will only escalate the situation. Any defense also heightens the anger of the client. If you are unsuccessful in calming the client, call for assistance.

- *Document everything.* Carefully document the entire episode completely. In doing so, remain neutral regarding your feelings. Describe the incident, what was said, and how you responded. Identify any actions taken to resolve the conflict. Be very careful not to use derogatory language in your documentation. It is not appropriate, for example, to say the client was "rude." State facts, not emotions.

Legal

- *If you find yourself feeling hostile toward clients, examine your feelings and discuss your response with someone who can help you sort through your reaction.* Continuous giving to others can drain you, but you must be relatively free of anxiety to be therapeutic.

Self-Awareness

- *Take a breather following an upsetting episode with a client.* Even a few minutes can help calm your own feelings and enable you to give full attention to your responsibilities. Take a coffee break, walk around the block if you can, perform some other task for a few moments. All of these examples can help to ease stress and anxiety.

THE AGGRESSIVE CLIENT

If conflict escalates beyond the angry state, clients may become aggressive and/or verbally abusive. In the opening case study, the verbal abuse occurs when the customer and the pharmacy assistant belittle each other and make threats. The pharmacy assistant's "Good riddance" statement while tossing the prescription back at the customer escalates the customer's anger into additional verbal abuse and aggression when she says to the pharmacist, "Fire that incompetent witch." "Case Study: An Aggressive Client" illustrates aggression that results from a far different cause.

Case Study: An Aggressive Client

Angel is 84 years old and resides in a memory care unit specifically designed for individuals with Alzheimer's disease. She does not wander, for the most part sticks to herself, and does not bother anyone. When her husband Pete comes to see her today, however, she shows alarm. Angel does not respond when he calls her by name. When he tries to put his arm around her and give her the lilacs he brought, she steps back, screams at him, and shouts, "Go away! Get out of my room! Who are you?" Pete is heartbroken. One of the nursing assistants observes this behavior and suggests Pete step outside into the hall. The assistant then assures Angel that it is okay. "There was a mistake, the man is gone now. Don't worry, you are safe." Angel calms down and goes to her rocking chair to look out the window. The nursing assistant suggests Pete go get a cup of coffee in the dining room and come back when he is finished because she believes Angel may be just fine by then. Pete goes for the coffee. When he comes back, he carefully approaches Angel in the rocking chair with a big grin and shows her the lilacs. She returns his smile and, with obvious pleasure, reaches for the lilacs and dips her face in their blossoms to smell the fragrance. Pete gently bends down to kiss his wife on the forehead.

As illustrated in "Case Study: An Aggressive Client," unfortunately, aggression is often exhibited in persons with Alzheimer's disease. Sometimes they kick, bite, grab, curse (although they may never have cursed when healthy), throw things, and scream. Of the more than 4.5 million Americans with Alzheimer's disease, half may show these behaviors. It is fairly common for a person with this disease to become aggressive with a family member they do not recognize or even believe their family is stealing from them. Generally, out-of-control frustration is the cause of aggressive behavior. Some individuals have an underlying aggression that only exhibits itself when control is lost. This kind of aggression usually is the result of unresolved anger and a loss of self-esteem. Some descriptors of people exhibiting aggression inappropriately include the following:

- Becoming suspicious of others over very small matters
- Joking at someone else's expense
- Confronting people with long, involved analyses of their behavior
- Becoming hostile, antagonistic, or resentful, or carrying a grudge
- Becoming uncooperative, caustic, sarcastic, rude, and critical
- Becoming demanding, complaining, and/or threatening
- Threatening to inflict or actually inflicting personal injury

Although you can do little about a client's unresolved anger, it may help to recognize that it may be a possible reason for aggression. Helping clients cope with anger and aggression is important. If aggression is turned inward on the self, the client may become depressed. Both children and adults need to be taught appropriate behavior for dealing with their anger.

In the case study with Angel, the nursing assistant demonstrated knowledge and skill in asking Pete to wait in the hall while she calmed Angel. Having Pete wait a little bit before he again approached Angel was a perfect response. When Pete returned, Angel no longer had any recollection of the earlier encounter and fear.

Sometimes it is difficult to know when conflict may turn to aggression and verbal abuse, but it is for certain that, when anger is not diminished and the conflict intensifies, aggression and verbal abuse are likely to follow. It may help to remember that expressions of anger and aggression move through a process illustrated below:

Physical or Emotional STRESSOR

↓

Painful FEELINGS

↓

ANGER

↓

ACTING OUT

The customer in the pharmacy was stressed because she had to wait in the doctor's office and she feared the possibility of missing an important engagement. She is likely feeling inadequate, since she believes she will fail to make the appointment. This is a painful feeling. These feelings lead to the statements that express frustration. The pharmacy assistant may not have encountered someone like this before, but feels responsible for "fixing" the problem. (A good question to ask in such a situation is, "Is it my responsibility to 'fix' this problem?")

Trigger words or statements are a response to the painful feelings. Triggers come from one's own values, beliefs, or expectations about how things should be. Anger follows, then acting out.

The Therapeutic Response

Professionalism

The guidelines for a therapeutic response to clients who are angry are also important to remember for clients who are aggressive. It is always better to try to resolve the conflict, placing yourself in the shoes of the other person to understand his or her needs and frustration, yet protecting yourself as necessary. Setting personal limits is helpful. "I can call another pharmacy with this prescription for you, if you cannot wait a few moments. Otherwise, I will ask you to leave if you continue to swear at me and make threats." This kind of statement alerts the offender that the limit has been reached. Often the offender will become embarrassed and retreat rather quickly. Then an agreeable solution is quite possible.

If the client continues to threaten and the anger increases, protect yourself. "I cannot accommodate your needs. Please leave the pharmacy now." Most individuals will leave. If not, make certain you have an escape route. Move yourself closer to the door. Call for assistance. This action may shock the aggressor into quieting down. If Angel's aggression in the case study had elevated further, it might have been best for the nursing assistant to make certain Angel was safe, then retreat from the room and close the door if necessary. She could then explain to Pete that Angel did not recognize him but that if he comes back tomorrow, it will probably be just fine.

Self-Awareness

As a helping professional, you must remember that you chose this profession. You made a conscious decision to serve people. You enter daily into relationships with your clients that are nonreciprocal. If clients become angry and belittle you, you do not have the right to belittle them back. You have the right not to lose your self-respect, but you do not have

(continues)

The Therapeutic Response   (*Continued*)

the right to disrespect your clients. You must always remember that your client is worthy of respect, no matter how wrong he or she is. The respect you give your clients is not dependent upon their achievements or lessened by their inappropriate behavior.

With those thoughts in mind, the best way to respond to angry, aggressive, and abusive clients is to listen empathically, show respect for others and yourself, remember not to take the event personally, and communicate assertively as necessary. Do not let someone else's bad day ruin yours. Learn how to short-circuit the anger process. Consider the following statements as possibilities:

- "It must be frustrating to have to wait, first for the doctor, and now for the pharmacist."
- "While I cannot fill this prescription for you, I can hasten the process by getting everything started for the pharmacist. Do you have insurance? Is this a medication you have taken before?"
- "Here's the pharmacist now. I will tell him you are in a hurry."
- "Would you like to use our phone to call your appointment while we get the medication ready?"
- "Thanks for choosing our pharmacy. I hope your afternoon goes a little more smoothly."

ABUSED OR ABUSIVE CLIENTS

Case Study: An Abused Client

Sam is brought to the medical clinic by his granddaughter and primary caregiver, Rebecca. Rebecca always comes with her grandfather, but seems agitated and nervous on this visit. Sam is suffering from the first stages of senile dementia. In the examination room, as the medical assistant rolls up Sam's sleeve to take his blood pressure, she sees large black and blue blotches on his skin. She asks, "Sam, what happened here?" Sam replies in a whisper, "Rebecca hits me when I soil the bed."

Stop and Consider 7.2

Before reading further, gather your thoughts about abuse and abusive relationships.

1. What have you heard about abuse in health care settings?

2. Have you known someone in a relationship that is abusive? What did you do?

3. How do you feel about someone who abuses another?

4. Have you ever been so angry that you wanted to hurt someone? If so, what helped to calm your anger?

In the previous section, you learned about how anger is processed and how it escalates. Turn your attention now to abusive behavior that is acted out toward individuals—many times in the family setting, and often to those who are powerless to change the actions of the abuser. This type of abuse may be emotional, physical (Figure 7-1), or sexual. Abusive behavior may come from friends and acquaintances, family members, and less often, strangers. Sadly, it may also come from overworked and untrained health care workers. Behavior is *violent* when there is intent to do harm. This harm may be in the form of emotional abuse, which is at first less obvious than physical or sexual abuse. In general, abuse is usually the result of biological, psychological, social, and cultural factors.

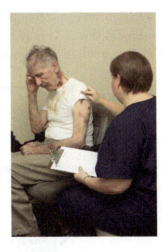

FIGURE 7-1   The medical assistant notices bruises on an older adult's arms.

Abusers usually suffer from low self-esteem and feelings of powerlessness, and blame others for their actions. They are also angry and frustrated. Without a feeling of self-worth, it is difficult to be confident and assertive; therefore, people with low self-esteem and a lack of confidence have a difficult time maintaining close and intimate relationships. They often feel threatened. Violence becomes a way to gain power and control over others.

Abusers are manipulators and easily rationalize and minimize their abusive behavior. They find it much easier to blame others for their abusive behavior than to accept responsibility for themselves. Abuse most often occurs when people have not been able to control their feelings of frustration and anger. The smallest event can trigger an abusive episode. The people closest to the abuser at this time usually become the abuser's target.

PHASES OF VIOLENCE

Violence has been identified in a number of ways, but the three phases of violence most often used to describe abuse are (1) the tension-building phase, (2) the crisis phase when abuse occurs, and (3) the calm or honeymoon phase (Figure 7-2). These phases may vary depending upon the individuals and the particular circumstances; sometimes the phases do not exist at all. When they do exist in an abusive situation, the phases are likely to become shorter, more violent, more frequent, and increasingly unpredictable over time.

Tension-Building Phase

There may be a triggering event that precipitates this phase. Tension builds; communication breaks down. It may be the 4-year-old spilling milk all over the dinner table or an adult getting into a "fender-bender." Perhaps it occurs

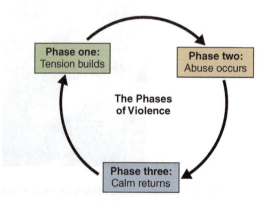

FIGURE 7-2   The phases of violence.

when a resident in a nursing facility refuses important medications and is rude to the caregiver. The abuser begins to lose control and humiliates the abused with verbal attacks. The abused often tries to placate or appease the abuser in order to cope. As the verbal assaults continue, threats are made. Pushing or slapping may occur. The abused will try to avoid the abuse; the abuser blames the abused for the situation. The abused often becomes detached emotionally and psychologically as the abuser increases control and possessiveness.

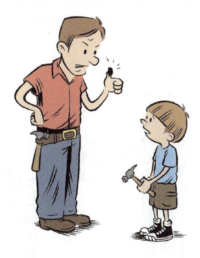

"CAN'T YOU DO ANYTHING RIGHT?"

Crisis Phase (Abuse Incident)

As anxiety reaches a climax, the abuser is very unpredictable; a series of "minor" assaults may occur over a period of time, or there may be very serious injury from a major assault. Death can even result. This phase may last just minutes or several hours. The abuser may isolate or lock up the victim. The abused is traumatized, will try to adapt in order to survive, and may even escape or hide, but usually returns after the crisis is over. Many times, the return to the environment where the abuse took place is because there is no place else to go.

Calm or Honeymoon Phase

The abuse ceases. The abuser promises to change, may ask for forgiveness, and be very loving; however, the abuser will continue to blame the abused. Both the abuser and the abused are relieved the crisis is past. Both may be emotionally and physically exhausted. The abused wants to believe that the violence will not happen again and often minimizes the abuse. In the case study at the beginning of this section, Sam's willingness to speak out about his bruises is very courageous. Remember never to belittle such a statement and to help someone like Sam feel safe and protected regarding his revelation.

In the health care setting such as a nursing facility, the abuser most likely makes the abused feel totally at fault and may threaten additional harm if any mention is made of the abuse or transgression. This harm may come in the form of denied privileges, medications kept from the abused, and denial of food or attention to comfort.

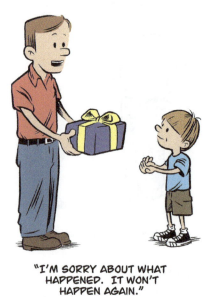

"I'M SORRY ABOUT WHAT HAPPENED. IT WON'T HAPPEN AGAIN."

TYPES OF ABUSE AND VIOLENCE

Four types of abuse are covered in this chapter. They are intimate partner violence (IPV), child abuse, abuse of older adults, and rape. At one time or another, all health care professionals will be faced with the challenge of communicating therapeutically with both the abusers and the survivors of such abuse.

Intimate Partner Violence

Intimate partner violence (IPV) is defined by the Centers for Disease Control and Prevention (CDC) as physical, sexual, or psychological/emotional violence directed toward a spouse or former spouse, current or former partner, or current or former dating partner. IPV refers to abuse between married people or people in an intimate heterosexual or same-sex relationship. The term *domestic violence* may be used also; however, IPV defines the broader scope of the problem. The abuser may be either male or female. The CDC adds stalking to the definition of IPV.

Stalking is the repeated behavior that causes individuals a high level of fear, and may refer to actions such as spying, pursuing, and threatening. The CDC reported in 2014 that 20 persons per minute are victims of IPV. Equal numbers of women and men reported being stalked prior to age 25.

The violence described in the CDC's definition of IPV fits in other areas of abuse also, but is further defined here.

Physical Violence

This type of abuse uses physical force with the intent to do harm. There is the potential for injury, disability, and even death. Physical violence includes, but is not limited to, choking, shaking, throwing, pushing, scratching, punching, burning, using a weapon, restraining, and using one's body size and strength against another.

Sexual Violence

Sexual violence includes (1) forcing a person to engage in a sexual act against his or her will, even if the act is not completed; (2) attempting or completing a sexual act with an individual who is unable or incapable of understanding or declining participation in the act because of disability, the influence of alcohol or drugs, or intimidation; and (3) abusive sexual contact.

Psychological/Emotional Violence

This type of abuse may include, but is not limited to, humiliation and control, isolation from friends and family, withholding of information, deliberate embarrassment or diminishment of an individual, and denial of access to resources.

The last decade has seen an increase in reports of IPV. Survivors of this type of abuse often report living in relationships characterized by fear, anger, and frustration. Wife battering is most commonly reported, but husband battering is on the rise. Women may receive more serious injuries since, generally, they have less physical strength than men, but women are more likely to use a weapon when they abuse.

Cultural

⊕ In some cultures women continue to be viewed as property—first of their fathers, then of their spouses. This patriarchal authority, still supported by some religions and cultures, leads some men to believe that their wives must submit to their authority or be disciplined by them. Abused women often rationalize that their abuse is caused by their own behavior and their own worthlessness. A person who leaves an abusive relationship or divorces the abuser still mourns the death of the abusive relationship. To obtain emotional health, this individual may need to work through the grieving process.

Child Abuse

Child abuse is evidence of parental/caregiver frustration, anger, and inability to fulfill parental obligations. Some parents and caregivers envision a fine line between discipline and abuse, and child abuse statistics are inadequate in describing the problem. Many individuals are reluctant to report child abuse even when mandated to do so by law. Few family members will admit to abusing or neglecting their children, and children usually do not admit they have been abused. Many think the actions against them are normal or are the result of some wrong they have committed. Children's sense of self comes from the parents or primary caregivers who are abusing them.

Legal

The 1990 Victims of Child Abuse Act (reauthorized for funding in 2014) defines abuse and neglect in the following terms: *Child abuse* refers to the deliberate harm or injury of a child by a parent or caregiver. *Negligence* occurs when a parent or caregiver fails to provide the basic necessities for life. *Physical injury* refers to serious bodily harm, severe bruising, lacerations, fractures, and internal injury. *Mental injury* includes harm to a child's psychological or intellectual well-being. *Sexual abuse* involves coercing a child into sexually implicit conduct, including molestation, rape, prostitution, or any form of sexual exploitation. *Sexually explicit conduct* is actual or simulated sexual intercourse, masturbation, lustful exhibition of the genitals, or sexual gratification from inflicting pain on others. *Child molestation* involves oral-genital contact, genital fondling or viewing, and masturbation. *Sexual exploitation* is child prostitution or pornography where sexually explicit reproductions of a child's image are used. *Incest* refers to sexual relations between children and blood relatives or family members.

People who abuse children sexually often were sexually abused themselves. Abusers may begin to abuse in their teens. If discovered, the excuse of experimentation will often dismiss their offenses. Most sexual abusers will repeat the behavior throughout their lives, even when caught and punished or given treatment. There is no reliable method of changing the behavior of people who sexually abuse children.

The close parent–child or primary caregiver–child relationship often confuses health care professionals trying to make a diagnosis, since both parties will exhibit deep concern for each other. Parents or caregivers who bring abused children in for treatment are often careful never to use the same clinic twice, and always have an explanation for the injuries.

Abuse of Older Adults

Abuse of older adults is defined as the harm or neglect that is inflicted upon someone who is 60 years of age or older. Abuse of older adults is more underreported than child abuse. Identifying abuse of older adults is difficult unless there is outright battering. Even then, excuses are likely offered. Abused older adults rarely report violence toward them, mostly because they fear loss of a living arrangement or retaliation. Older adults are also ashamed that someone they may have nurtured in childhood is now abusing them.

Abuse of older adults most likely occurs in two locations: (1) in the home or primary living residence of the older adult (domestic abuse), and (2) in a nursing home or some type of long-term care facility (institutional abuse). Abuse of older adults occurs in many different forms:

- *Physical abuse* is identified as threats or harm that result in injury, impairment, or pain. Physical abuse includes, but is not limited to, beating, whipping, slapping, pushing, shoving, shaking, kicking, pinching, force-feeding, inappropriate use of drugs or restraints, and any rough handling.

- *Psychological/emotional abuse* occurs when there is a lack of basic emotional support, respect, and love. This type of abuse includes name-calling, verbal assaults, and dehumanizing the older adult. It may include isolating the person from family and friends, threatening to punish, intimidating, treating the older person like a child, and terrorizing.

- *Neglect or abandonment* consists of confinement, denial of essential needs, or isolation. The neglected older adult may lack the necessities of food, water, shelter, clothing, medicine, warmth, and safety. Individuals may not have adequate assistance with bathing, be physically restrained, lack assistance in moving around their environment, and have lack of access to supplies for incontinence. Abandonment occurs when a caregiver deserts a vulnerable older adult.

- *Sexual abuse* is sexual contact without consent. Sexual abuse may include kissing, fondling, or touching of the genitals or making the older adult fondle someone else's genitals. Sexual assault or forcing the older adult to observe sexual acts or pornographic material is sexual abuse. Telling "dirty" stories, spying on them in the bathroom, and forcing nudity upon them is sexual abuse.

- *Financial exploitation* is the use of finances, property, or anything of value belonging to the older adult in an illegal or improper manner. Any misuse of the older adult's money or belongings—such as withholding Social Security checks, using a charge card without permission, scamming or tricking the elder person into withdrawing money from the bank and then taking the money, stealing household goods or valuables, forcing an older adult to alter a will to benefit the abuser, and forging the older adult's signature— is considered financial exploitation or abuse.

- *Violation of rights* includes denial of adequate medical care, taking property without due process, not allowing the older adult to attend religious services of his or her choice, and taking away a person's right to make his or her own decisions while still competent to do so.

Institutional abuse of older adults may occur in any of the forms just described. There are other violations, however, that may occur in a long-term care setting. The use of physical restraints may be necessary on rare occasions; however, when restraints are applied against an older adult's will or the wishes of family members because of understaffing or lack of training, or when the staff is too busy to pay adequate attention to an older adult, institutional abuse occurs. Other forms of institutional abuse are over- or under-medicating, force-feeding, rough handling while moving the older adult or giving medications or treatment, ignoring pleas of help, improper hand washing by health care providers, inadequate attention to changing diapers or disposable briefs, failing to provide adequate psychological care or stimulation, overcharging or double-billing for medical or personal services, and stealing personal property or money.

Caregivers in nursing homes and long-term care facilities may be inadequately educated, trained, and prepared for the task. Often they are not comfortable with the language or culture of the older adult, and if serious disease or dementia is involved, it is far less stressful to treat the older adult as a nonperson. It is fairly easy to provide simple care for older adults, but it can become far less pleasant if the caregiver must feed, bathe, and provide assistance in the bathroom. If the older adult is appreciative of the care and is able to communicate, the caregiving is made easier. If the older adult is aggressive, even violent, the caregiver will be more stressed, and may struggle to remain professional at all times and in all situations.

Caregiving in the home is very stressful also. Caregivers may be overburdened with the responsibility of caring for an older adult. This may cause the caregiver to ignore the basic needs of the older adult. Often, younger caregivers do not understand the social needs of older adults. They do not realize that the losses (significant other, driver's license, physical health, etc.) suffered by older adults precipitate grief. The despair, complaints, and criticism expressed by older adults who are grieving may become difficult for the caregiver to understand or tolerate.

Psychological and physical changes associated with aging may cause some older adults to withdraw from social activities. Caregivers may tire of sitting and listening to these individuals. They assume the role of parent and assign the role of child to the older adult. This role reversal discourages the older adult's independence and integrity.

Rape

Rape is forcible sexual intercourse with an unwilling partner. The rape incident may include **sodomy**. Rape is not a sexual act; it is an act of violence. No person invites rape, either by behavior or dress. Rape may include more than one person or more than two, as seen in gang rape. Criminal sexual assault is identified as penetration of any part of the abuser's body with any object, using force and without consent. Anyone can be raped: infants, older adults, those who are lesbian or gay, people with disabilities, and individuals of every ethnic, social, religious, and cultural background. While the majority of rape is committed against women and girls, men and boys are raped also. Men and boys are also often attacked by gangs and are assaulted with weapons. Bullying that includes physical assault often becomes rape.

Law enforcement personnel and many legal professionals refer to the individual who has been raped as a "victim." Most health care professionals and social service professionals refer to the individual who has been raped or abused as a "survivor." Words and their meanings are very powerful. Both words are used in this text.

Health care professionals may find it helpful to recognize that rapists are generally identified in three categories: angry, power, and sadistic. The *angry rapist* displaces anger to the abused, uses a fair amount of physical force, and degrades the victim by forcing oral sex or masturbation.

The angry rapist may urinate on the victim. The angry rapist most often preys on someone who is older or vulnerable.

The *power rapist* is the most common type, and uses only the amount of force necessary to subdue the victim. The power rapist is seeking power and control and often intimidates the victim. The power rapist may fantasize that the victim is sexually attracted to the rapist, wants to know if the victim "is enjoying this," and may ask to see the victim again after the rape.

The *sadistic rapist*, the least common type, seeks sexual gratification as an outlet for aggression. Sexuality and aggression go hand in hand. This rapist is aroused by the victim's death, and may achieve orgasm at that moment. Penetration may be obtained with an instrument. The rapist may have intercourse with the victim after death.

Survivors of rape generally experience four distinct crisis stages in their recovery. They are as follows:

- The first phase is one of shock, disbelief, and fear. This phase can last for 2–3 weeks in some cases.

- The second phase is a time of adjustment. The survivor may appear outwardly to be doing fine, but inwardly is in denial of the entire event.

- The third phase is a time of depression, self-doubt, and the need to talk about the rape. Often, the survivor has difficulty sleeping and is quite anxious.

- The fourth phase is a time of recovery, with the recognition that the blame lays totally with the abuser rather than the survivor. The survivor begins to trust others again and feel comfortable in daily activities.

Like any experience that may be described in phases or stages, survivors do not necessarily go through all the stages in a given pattern. They may go through the phases many times, or may never move out of one phase. How clients cope is dependent upon factors such as how others react to the event, their own personal development, and their willingness to participate in crisis counseling. The latter allows the opportunity for support and the ability to discharge the shame, guilt, and anger felt over the event.

INDICATORS OF ABUSE

Emotional abuse is often not evident until many years later. Emotional abuse usually takes its toll in long-lasting physical or psychological problems and is difficult for health care professionals to diagnose. However, health care professionals will want to be alert to those who are often extremely punitive in their treatment of others, who are aggressive and verbally abusive to others, and who are easily threatened by others or exhibit a low self-esteem. Individuals who have been abused typically have few defense mechanisms for coping with anxiety and stress. Health care professionals can and should provide resources to help them learn to control their abusive behavior.

Physical abuse may be observed by health care professionals when survivors seek medical attention or are brought to health care facilities by family or friends. Burns, bruises, lacerations, broken bones, malnutrition—all are examples of what may be physical evidence of abuse. Special attention should be given to the individual who denies any form of abuse when the abuse seems obvious. It is important to provide survivors with information on how to keep safe, help survivors realize that they were not the cause of the abuse, and allow them their personal dignity.

Children who are physically abused will exhibit evidence of the abuse. X-rays may reveal fractures in various stages of healing. Burns, bruises, and lacerations are often apparent. Sexual abuse may be evidenced by difficulty in walking or sitting; torn, stained, or bloody underclothing; pain or itching in the genital area; bruises or bleeding in external genitalia, vaginal, anal, or mouth areas; and sexually transmitted diseases (especially in preteens) or pregnancy. If medical treatment is sought early enough, rape or sexual intercourse may be evidenced by the presence of semen. In some cases, there may be no obvious physical signs or symptoms.

Children who have an interest in or knowledge of sexual acts or language inappropriate to their age may have been sexually abused. These children may reenact sexual scenes with dolls, in drawing, or with friends. They may attempt to touch the genitals of adults, other children, or animals.

People who are physically abused may exhibit aggressive behavior, and children also may **regress** (Appendix B) to an earlier stage of development, such as wetting or soiling their underwear. Children may threaten their playmates or dolls. People may be aggressive toward animals, and anger is directed everywhere. Abused people often withdraw into a fantasy world. People may exhibit fear of specific places or people. Sleep disturbances and nightmares are common.

TREATMENT

Any abused individual coming to a health care facility must receive prompt treatment for any injuries. A rape kit must be done immediately in cases of rape. A rape kit is filled with little boxes, microscope slides, and plastic bags for collecting and storing evidence such as clothing fibers, hairs, saliva, or semen.

Legal

Samples of this evidence may be used in court. The circumstances and the place of treatment will determine if law enforcement is notified at that time. The survivor needs to feel safe and have a safe place to go. Provide a list of such places or other possible resources, and discuss alternatives. Focus on the survivor, not on the violent event. Underlying anxiety and anger needs to be assessed. The survivor needs acceptance and approval and is very vulnerable to any form of rejection, real or perceived. Eventually, survivors can be helped to confront the crisis and talk about their feelings. Help survivors identify effective coping behaviors to deal with the crisis. Community agencies may provide the best resources for this process.

Remember that abusers also need treatment. Health care professionals treating an abuser must be assured of a safe environment for themselves and the abuser. Observing the abuser's personal space is important, so as not to appear threatening. A violent person may have a personal space requirement up to four times larger than for a nonviolent person. Involve the abuser in therapy; it is helpful when the courts require therapy. The abuser must learn assertive, nonviolent ways of expressing anger and frustration and communicating with others. Try to communicate acceptance of the abuser's feelings but *not* acceptance of the violent behavior.

REPORTING AND DOCUMENTATION

Legal

All states have laws that identify specific requirements for reporting abuse (Figure 7-3). All 50 states mandate the reporting of child abuse. IPV is a criminal offense in most states, but not all require reporting unless

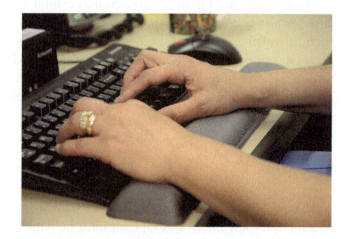

FIGURE 7-3   A provider documenting in a clinic medical record.

a weapon is used for the abuse. A majority of the 50 states have enacted legislation regarding abuse of older adults. It is not the purpose of this text to be a legal guide, since new laws are legislated almost daily; therefore, health care professionals must become knowledgeable of their state's requirements. Hospital and emergency room personnel are generally more equipped to report, document, and treat an abused individual than the ambulatory health care professionals. However, not all abused individuals present themselves to emergency rooms.

Each state has laws defining child abuse and mandating that suspected child abuse and neglect be reported. People most likely required to report suspected abuse and neglect include health care professionals, social service and law enforcement personnel, educators, and professional people working with children. Any person who believes that a child may be abused or neglected may report, in good faith, to law enforcement or child protection agencies. Such people are protected against liability as a result of making the report, provided there is reasonable cause to suspect child abuse or neglect. Reports may be made by telephone, in writing, or in person to the local law enforcement agency or appropriate state agency.

The most difficult circumstances may be when an abused older adult or a survivor of IPV asks that no report be made to law enforcement officials. If states do not have laws that mandate reporting the offense, protecting the survivor from further abuse may be the best approach. Make certain that these individuals have the telephone numbers of safe places to go and that they understand their options.

The health care records of survivors of violence and abuse will likely be used in a court of law. The medical record should not, therefore, include inferences or conclusions of the assault. Only facts should be reported. Those facts might include:

- History and account of the incident
- Words expressed by the client(s) and in quotations
- Photographs of injuries when possible
- Documentation, if known, of the extent of force that was used
- Specific, factual observations
- Objective findings and treatment established

Any evidence collected (body fluids, clothing, etc.) is to be bagged, labeled, and safely preserved and protected for law enforcement, making certain the "chain of evidence" is not broken. Anyone reporting the case should write down the information as clearly and completely as possible.

The Therapeutic Response

Professional

Some suggestions are made under "Treatment" (see pp. 181–182). Responding therapeutically in any circumstance involving violence and abuse is a challenge. It helps to concentrate on the individual seeking treatment and not on the violent act. Do not shame or ridicule. Be gentle, calm, and supportive. Give reassurance and offer explanations of the services and procedures. Be patient and do not rush interactions. Note the nonverbal as well as the verbal responses of the client. Ensure the client's safety, privacy, and prompt treatment. It is important to assist both the abuser *and* the abused to seek proper counseling. This may involve personal as well as family counseling. Parents Anonymous provides support for parents who have abused their children. There are support groups for IPV survivors and rape victims also. They include VOICES: Victims of Incest Can Emerge Survivors; RAINN: Rape Abuse Incest National Network; and a number of Web sites related to IPV available on the Internet.

Unless a trust relationship already exists between health care professionals and the abuser or the abused, it may be difficult to establish therapeutic communication.

It is interesting to note that survivors usually experience the same kinds of feelings as the abuser. Their self-esteem may be seriously damaged by the abusive situation. They feel powerless and often blame themselves. They feel ashamed, frustrated, and angry. They grieve the loss of their self-concept. Significant others and family members pose problems if they are not supportive and accepting of the victim. Health care professionals can assist family members and friends in understanding this dimension of abuse and recovery.

One of the goals in any of the violent situations identified is to protect survivors from any further abuse and to break the cycle of violence. Individuals may need temporary shelter. Always have a list of phone numbers available for such services. Encourage family members to seek counseling and treatment. Help potential abusers identify their tendency toward abuse and seek treatment. Provide appropriate rehabilitative and supportive services to high-risk families. Survivors of abuse can get caught in multiple social agencies that have differing goals. Clients easily become confused and even feel victimized again by the actions taken to protect their abuser. Encourage these clients to hold fast to their goals and continue the path to recovery.

UNDERSTANDING SELF

Self-Awareness

It is important for health care professionals to examine their own attitudes toward anger, aggression, abuse, and the abuser. Treating these clients with disgust, anger, and avoidance is not a therapeutic response. Stereotypes about individuals who are easy to anger, become aggressive, or inflict violence need careful self-assessment. Feeling frustrated and powerless to change situations of long-standing abuse can prevent a therapeutic response. A health care professional who lives in a household where anger and aggression is commonly expressed or who has witnessed abuse may have difficulty in remaining objective and being helpful to either the abuser or the abused. But the opposite also may be true. Health care professionals who have "traveled down the same path" may be the most therapeutic because they know what is and is not helpful.

It can be difficult to respond therapeutically to clients who are angry, or who get aggressive, even abusive, in their response to you as a health care professional, and it is even more difficult to respond therapeutically to the abusive client. Personal feelings that enter into the relationship cloud a professional's effectiveness unless they can be set aside.

SUMMARY

Professionalism

Health care professionals who are therapeutic realize that their roles may place them in circumstances that can be frightening, unpleasant, even revolting, and that they will be called upon to perform their duties with sensitivity and without judgment. Health care professionals who are successful in this task lead a balanced daily life and see the potential for good they can bring to all situations. They have learned how to set limits and how to be compassionate without emotional attachment, and they have learned to recognize their vulnerabilities. They understand the nonreciprocal relationship between client and health care provider.

EXERCISES

Exercise 1

1. Identify at least three resources in your community that would be appropriate for the client who may be experiencing aggressive behavioral patterns.

2. Do a little research on human trafficking, and identify how it might be related to the chapter content. Might you see survivors of this offense in a medical setting? If so, how should they be treated?

Exercise 2

Respond to the following situations:

1. Dick, a businessman who has been waiting for his appointment for 20 minutes, says, "I'll not wait another moment for the doctor. Please recommend another physician who can see me."
   You feel _____.
   You respond _____.

2. Sharon, a coworker, remarks to you, "Why do you always insist on making such a mess in the appointment schedule?"
   You feel _____.
   You respond _____.

3. You must tell the client who is smoking in the lobby that he cannot smoke in the hospital. How will you explain that policy?
   _____.

4. You know not all clients have easy veins for blood draws. Today, a regular client known to you jerks her arm as you begin the blood draw with the words, "Why in the world do you always make it hurt so much? Can't you make it easier? Next time, I'll ask for someone else."
   You feel _____.
   You respond _____.

Exercise 3

Select a character who is an abuser or a survivor of abuse in a novel, movie, or television program. What kind of behavior does this person exhibit? Write a short report with your response.

Exercise 4

Briefly describe what you would say and how you would respond to the following situations. These exercises can be used in small group settings, used as role-playing exercises, or can be completed independent of others.

1. Your spouse/significant other uses verbal abuse and inappropriate language when you are arguing.

I feel _____.
I would say _____.

2. Your date does not listen or respond when you say "no" and "stop" during hugging, kissing, and fondling.
I feel _____.
I would say _____.

3. A client makes suggestive remarks to you while you are taking an ECG.
I feel _____.
I would say _____.

4. Assume you have just been a victim of physical and sexual abuse.
I feel _____.
I would want health care professionals to say _____.
What would have to happen for you to feel like a survivor rather than a victim? _____.

5. Your daughter, age 7, tells you with tears in her eyes, "Uncle Phil touched me down there while he was taking care of me."
I feel _____.
I would say _____.
What will be your next step? _____.

REVIEW QUESTIONS

Multiple Choice

1. Isaiah denies his fear of growing older and suffering from debilitating arthritis by insisting on continuing his training for a marathon. What is the name for this defense mechanism?

   a. Regression   **c.** Suppression

   b. Rationalization   **d.** Panic

2. What are the feelings that can turn into anger?

   a. Defensiveness, suspicion, and tension

   b. Depression, avoidance, and repression

   c. Denial, compensation, and fear

   d. Frustration, annoyance, and fear

3. What are the three phases of violence?
   a. The calm phase, the trigger phase, and the crisis phase
   b. The tension phase, the crisis phase, and the calm phase
   c. The trigger phase, the tension phase, and the violent phase
   d. Tension-building phase, the abusive incident, and the crisis result

4. In what relationships can IPV occur?
   a. Between spouses, work colleagues, and parents
   b. Between parents, cousins, and teacher
   c. Between spouses or partners, heterosexual or same-sex relationships—current or present
   d. Only between current spouses or partners

5. When a PCP determines that child abuse is evident, what are the next steps to be taken?
   a. Call the police
   b. Make a referral to the nearest hospital
   c. Put the parent in a separate room, lock the door, and then call police
   d. Preserve evidence, protect the child, and call the appropriate authorities determined by state law

FOR FURTHER CONSIDERATION

1. Discuss with an acquaintance the use of the term *survivor* rather than *victim*. Can you identify circumstances where one term is preferred over the other?

2. Consider your actions/response if you believe there has been abuse of a client, but your provider/employer says, "Leave it alone. Don't get involved."

CASE STUDIES

Case Study 1

You are a certified nursing assistant sitting with another assistant at break time in the lounge. Your morning has been particularly frustrating, but you are surprised when your colleague blurts out, "I can handle the dementia people most of the time, but when they get mean, I get mean right back!"

1. What do you say? What do you do?

2. Identify any suggestions you might make to help your colleague.

Case Study 2

You are in a department store with your spouse and teenage son. You are all aware of a fairly noisy gentleman who approaches the counter, asking where he might find boys' pajamas. A woman who appears to be his wife and a young boy are with him. The man notices sweatshirts with humorous slogans on them. One woman's sweatshirt says, "The Queen Who Must Be Obeyed" on it. He jerks his son by the arm, points to the sweatshirt, and says, "We don't have that kind of b_ _ _ in our house, son, and you won't have that either!" The woman looks at you with pleading eyes, but shrugs her shoulders and walks away.

1. What kind of discussion might you have when your family returns to the car?

2. What information is important for your son to have?

REFERENCES AND RESOURCES

Centers for Disease Control and Prevention. (2014). *National intimate partner and sexual violence survey infographic (2014)*. Retrieved from www.cdc.gov/violenceprevention/nisvs/infographic.html.

Domestic and dating violence handbook (8th ed.). (2008). Seattle, WA: Metropolitan King County Council.

Frisch, N. C., & Frisch, L. E. (2010). *Psychiatric mental health nursing* (4th ed.). Clifton Park, NY: Cengage Learning.

Lewis, M. A., Tamparo, C. D., & Tatro, B. (2012). *Medical law, ethics, and bioethics* (7th ed.). Philadelphia: F. A. Davis.

Saltzman, L. E., Panslow, J. L., McMahon, P. M., & Shelly, G. A. (2002). *Intimate partner violence, surveillance: Uniform definitions and recommended data elements (version 1.0)*. Atlanta, GA: Centers for Disease Control and Prevention, National Center for Injury Prevention and Control.

Tamparo, C. D. (2016). *Diseases of the human body* (6th ed.). Philadelphia: F. A. Davis.

Chapter 8

The Therapeutic Response to Depressed and/or Suicidal Clients

CHAPTER OBJECTIVES

After completing this chapter, the learner should be able to:

- Define the key terms as presented in the glossary.

- Recognize the differences between the following types of depression: major and minor depression, persistent depressive disorder, reactive depression, bipolar disorder, major depression with seasonal pattern disorder, major depression disorder with peripartum-onset depression, and psychotic depression.

- Summarize the impacts of depression upon the life span.

- Illustrate therapeutic responses to depressed clients in each age group.

- Identify the high-risk groups for suicide.

- List the steps and stages involved in contemplating suicide.

- Describe the verbal and nonverbal messages sent by suicidal people.

- List criteria used to evaluate suicide potential.

- Illustrate therapeutic responses to the suicidal person.

Opening Case Study

Recently Jody, a 15-year-old, has not been acting like herself. She used to hang out with her friends after school; now when she comes home, she goes straight to her bedroom or stares at the television for hours. Jody was a very good student; however, her teachers report that she does not turn in assignments on time and her test scores are dropping. When asked about this, Jody responds, "I don't care. What's the point of it all?" When her friends call, she does not want to talk with them. She was active in her church youth group, but now is not interested in participating in those activities. She seems tired and listless and has lost noticeable weight. When her parents try to talk to her about what is wrong or how she feels, she gets irritable and snaps at them. She seems angry with them for expressing concern. Jody states, "I can't do anything right. Everything is hopeless and I'm worthless. Why bother?" This has been going on for several months, and her parents wonder if something is seriously wrong.

Stop and Consider 8.1

1. What signals is Jody sending that might cause her parents to be concerned?

2. What would trouble you as a parent the most?

INTRODUCTION

Depression has been described as feelings of despair, gloom, or emptiness; a sense of foreboding, numbness, hopelessness, or agony; or a negative sense of self-worth. Anyone can experience depression, and it can be brought on by a number of different causes. People may become depressed when their feeling of well-being is challenged or when they experience a loss of some type. Others experience depression because of unpleasant feelings, including sadness, boredom, apathy, even anger. Depression isn't a weakness, nor is it something that simply goes away. It can be treated with medication and psychological counseling; however, long-term treatment may be required for some types of depression.

Depression is a mood disorder that causes a persistent feeling of sadness and loss of interest (Figure 8-1). There is no diagnostic test for depression,

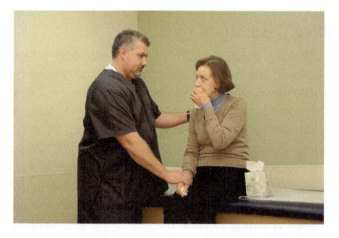

FIGURE 8-1   Depression doesn't just go away, but treatment options have a good success rate.

such as a blood test, urinalysis, or a scan, which is able to confirm whether someone has the illness. In the past, psychiatrists used different criteria to diagnose depression. With the advent of internationally recognized sets of diagnostic criteria such as the **Diagnostic and Statistical Manual of Mental Disorders, Fifth Edition (DSM-5)** and the **International Classification of Disease, 10 Clinical Modification (ICD-10-CM)**, much confusion has been alleviated. These criteria have led to a greater uniformity in approaches to the diagnosis and classification of depressive illnesses. The criteria and the classes of depression are continually updated with each new revision of DSM and ICD-CM, and there continue to be differences in opinion regarding criteria and classification among psychiatrists.

TYPES OF DEPRESSION

There are two types of depression: major and minor. According to the National Institute of Mental Health (NIMH) 20–25% of the U.S. adult population may experience a major depressive episode during their lifetime. Major depression, also known as clinical depression, affects how the client feels, thinks, and behaves, and can lead to a variety of emotional and physical problems. The client may have trouble doing normal day-to-day activities, and may feel as if life isn't worth living. Suicide is a very serious concern for these clients. Often symptoms are worse in the mornings but may last most of the day. Some clients may experience major depression only once in their lifetime while others may experience it several times. Major depression affects all ages, racial and ethnic populations, and gender groups.

Minor depression is a lesser form of clinical depression. Clients must have one of two symptoms for at least 2 weeks lasting most of the day and occurring nearly every day. The two symptoms are depressed mood and loss of interest or pleasure in things normally enjoyed. Additional criteria used to diagnose minor depression include symptoms that impact ability to function, symptoms that are not due to substance abuse or to a recent loss of a loved one, and having no history of a major depressive or manic episode. Table 8-1 lists some of the signs and symptoms that may be associated with depression in general. A client may not have all of the signs and symptoms listed but may still be diagnosed with depression.

Subclassifications of depression called specifiers are attached to the diagnosis. Table 8-2 indicates symptoms associated with each specifier.

Persistent Depressive Disorder

Persistent depressive disorder, formerly known as dysthymic disorder, was updated and renamed in DSM-5. Persistent depressive disorder is a less severe form of minor depression. Clients with this disorder still feel good and can function fairly well. Providers will want to evaluate the symptoms to be sure they are not caused by some physical condition

TABLE 8-1   **Signs and Symptoms of Depression**

- Feeling sad and unhappy
- Anger management issues
- Loss of interest or response to previously enjoyable events (loss of sex drive)
- Sleep disturbance
- Increase or decrease in appetite
- Anxiety
- Sluggishness
- Feelings of guilt
- Concentration problems
- Poor memory
- Difficulty making decisions
- Suicidal thoughts or attempts
- Unsupported medical symptoms

TABLE 8-2   **Signs and Symptoms Associated with Depression Specifiers**

Specifier	Characteristics
Anxious distress	Restlessness, irrational worry, loss of self-control
Mixed features	Depression with elevated self-esteem, excessive talking, racing thoughts
Melancholic features	Severe depression, lack of response to previously enjoyable events, early riser and bad mood, appetite changes, guilt, agitation, or sluggishness
Atypical features	Cheered by happy events, good appetite, sensitive to rejection, sleeps little, sluggish
Psychotic features	Depression coupled with delusions or hallucinations
Catatonia	Uncontrolled movement or body inflexibility
Peripartum onset	Depression occurring during or after pregnancy
Seasonal pattern	Depression related to changing seasons or seasonal lack of sunlight

such as hypothyroidism. In some cases major depression may precede persistent depressive disorder and a major depressive episode may even occur during persistent depressive disorder episodes. When the two depressions are experienced at the same time, it is termed double depression.

A combination of treatment options is available. One option is psychotherapy or talk therapy. During talk sessions clients will be encouraged to talk about their feelings. The listening provider can help the client establish realistic goals early on as the focus of therapy instead of focusing on the client's mood state. Appropriate coping skills to reduce stress for dealing with everyday life can be presented. Antidepressant medications may be used in combination with psychotherapy. It is important to remember that antidepressants may take several weeks to work fully. It may also take several weeks to safely discontinue an antidepressant.

Reactive Depression

Reactive depression is also referred to as an adjustment disorder with depressed mood. It is considered the most temporary form of minor depression and often follows the loss/death of a family member, a divorce, loss of a job, or not getting an anticipated promotion. *Loss* is the key. The loss may also include the loss of love, beauty, a home—loss of anything with meaning to the individual.

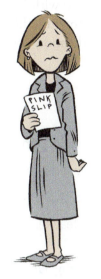

"THIS IS REALLY DEPRESSING."

Individuals suffering from reactive depression generally are able to work through the emotional distress for themselves by developing coping strategies to reduce stress associated with the loss. Medications are not recommended, since time seems to reduce the symptoms. Family and friends can be a big support, as they may be aware of the precipitating factor.

Bipolar Disorder (BPD)

Bipolar disorder (BPD), a type of major depression also known as manic-depressive disorder, alternates between the extreme highs of **mania** and severe lows or **hypomania**. Bipolar I disorder is classified as experiencing at least one manic episode with or without previous episodes of depression. Bipolar II clients experience at least one episode of depression and at least one hypomanic episode. According to DMS-5, the main difference between mania and hypomania is the degree of severity as well as an absence of **psychosis** in hypomania.

BPD tends to be familial but may also be caused by environmental factors. When discrete mood episodes happen four or more times per year the process is termed *rapid cycling*. Severe mania may require hospitalization primarily because of risky behaviors, suicidal thoughts, or psychotic symptoms such as delusions, hallucinations, and disorganized thinking.

BPD treatment includes medication and psychotherapy. Psychotherapy helps clients cope with the cyclical nature of the disease and can lead to better compliance with bipolar disorder medication. There is no cure for BPD and treatment is lifelong. Monitoring on a regular basis is required to ensure medication dosage is correct and that it is being taken as prescribed.

Stop and Consider   8.2

Review the opening case study about Jody and respond to the following questions:

1. List Jody's emotional symptoms of depression.

2. List Jody's physical symptoms of depression.

3. What action might her parents, teachers, and friends take?

Major Depressive Disorder with Seasonal Pattern Disorder

As the winter months progress, daylight hours grow shorter and winter storms fill the skies with dark clouds. These conditions will likely be severe for those who live in the northern parts of the world. Each year the decreased sunlight impacts 10–20% of people in the United States, causing seasonal pattern disorder.

Clients experiencing seasonal pattern disorder often complain of having less energy, trouble concentrating and fatigue, greater appetite with cravings for carbohydrates, weight gain, and a greater need for sleep. Females are at a higher risk for this disorder; however, men may experience more severe symptoms. Young people are more at risk than the older population. Seasonal pattern disorder has familial tendencies and often the client has experienced other types of depressions.

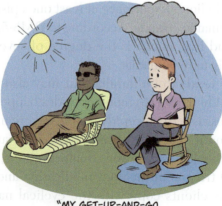

"MY GET-UP-AND-GO
GOT UP AND WENT."

Light therapy or phototherapy has become the treatment of choice for clients with seasonal pattern disorder. These individuals should get as much natural sunlight as possible. They may need to trim the bushes around windows or keep curtains and blinds open to allow more light to enter rooms. They should be encouraged to take walks and to consider taking part or all of their vacation during the winter visiting sunny areas of the country. As soon as spring arrives, the symptoms disappear.

Major Depression Disorder with Peripartum Onset (PPND)

Previously known as postpartum or paternal postnatal depression, PPND is a severe form of "baby blues" lasting anywhere from 3 months to 1 year. Stress seems to be one of several contributing factors to this type of depression. A new mother can feel overwhelmed with the responsibilities involved with caring for an infant. Sleepless nights, a colicky baby, illness, and lack of physical and emotional support for the new mom all add stress to this new family unit. When one adds the additional factor of fluctuating hormones and their role in peripartum depression, it is little wonder that many women experience this disorder (Figure 8-2).

Some mothers are afraid to admit they are depressed for fear of being deemed unfit or unable to care for the infant and perhaps losing the baby to social services. Support groups can play a major role in recovery. Sometimes

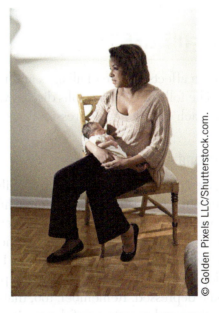

© Golden Pixels LLC/Shutterstock.com.

FIGURE 8-2   Approximately 14% of new mothers develop PPND.

just knowing that others also experience similar problems seems to be therapeutic. Physical and emotional support for an entire family can be found in support groups. Signs and symptoms of PPND frequently occur a few days after giving birth and include most of the symptoms found with other types of depression. Women suffering from PPND frequently have experienced previous episodes of depression, and may have had a miscarriage or lost an infant. Drug therapy can be helpful in some cases; however, caution must be used with any type of medication prescribed. Many medications enter the breast milk of nursing mothers and are passed on to their baby.

Psychotic Depression

Psychotic depression is a subtype of major depression. According to the National Institute of Mental Health, a person suffering from this type of depression is out of touch with reality. They may hear voices or experience strange and illogical ideas. Psychotic depression affects approximately one out of every four people admitted to the hospital for depression. The disorder is serious and clients may be at risk of suicide.

Treatment for psychotic depression is usually given in a hospital setting. Clients are closely monitored by mental health professionals. A variety of medications are used to stabilize the client's mood and may include a combination of antidepressants and antipsychotic drugs. These treatment approaches are quite effective; however, continual follow-up may be necessary.

DEPRESSION AND THE LIFE SPAN

Depression affects people of all ages and racial, ethnic, and socioeconomic groups. The following paragraphs discuss various age groups and the different ways each experience depression.

Children and Adolescents

At any given point in time, about 5% of children and adolescents in the general population suffer from depression. Children who are under stress, who experience loss, or who have attentional, learning, conduct, or anxiety disorders are at a higher risk for depression. Some researchers suggest that stresses are dealt with differently by boys and girls. For example, boys are more likely to develop behavioral and substance abuse problems, while girls are more apt to become depressed. Remember, too, that some depressions are familial.

The signs and symptoms of depression in children and adolescents are the same as for adults. Many times symptoms of depression are overlooked as normal behaviors or are misdiagnosed for disorders such as attention-deficit disorder (ADA) and attention-deficit/hyperactivity disorder (ADHD). According to child development experts, depressive behaviors lasting beyond 2 weeks should be investigated.

Bullying can also lead to depression and increases the risk of suicide in children and adolescents. Bullying is defined as unwanted, aggressive behavior that involves a real or perceived threat. The behavior is usually repeated over a period of time and may take place face-to-face or through social media. Bullying includes actions such as making threats, spreading rumors, attacking someone physically or verbally, and excluding someone from a group on purpose.

Early diagnosis and treatment for depression in children and adolescents are essential. Individual and family therapy is often helpful. **Cognitive-behavioral therapy (CBT)** and **interpersonal psychotherapy (IPT)** may be used to treat children and adolescents diagnosed with depression. Antidepressants may also be recommended as part of the treatment plan.

Adults

Women are almost twice as likely as men to experience both major and minor depression. This ratio does not seem to be influenced by racial and ethnic background or economic status. About half of the adults who are depressed believe depression is a personal weakness and are too embarrassed to seek help. Women are more likely to admit to feelings of depression and seek professional help. Men, more often than not, are socially conditioned to deny these feelings and to bury them. Repressing feelings can result in violent behavior directed both inwardly and outwardly. Facing discrimination regularly from society at large, and sometimes from family, coworkers, or classmates may create a higher risk for depression among the lesbian, gay, bisexual, and transgender (LGBT) population. This group may also experience an increase in illness, suicide, and homicide.

Older Adults

Older adults do not adapt to change as readily as younger individuals. Often, older adults are isolated from family and friends, who do not live nearby. They have experienced more loss and grief than other age groups. Previous coping methods used by individuals will have a direct impact on the individual's ability to adapt and accept change. Major depressions can affect older adults; however, it frequently goes undiagnosed and untreated. Often, the older adult experiences depression over a longer period of time and is accompanied by other medical illnesses and disabilities. Older adults who seem depressed can benefit from a medical workup and reassurance that depression is an illness and is fairly easily treated. Do not delay treatment until the older person begins to discuss suicide. Compared with younger people, older adults talk about killing themselves less, but are more successful at the attempts. The suicide rate in people age 80–84 is more than twice that of the general population. The National Institute of Mental Health considers depression in adults age 65 or older to be a major public health issue.

The Therapeutic Response

Individuals experiencing the effects of depression must have an environment that makes them feel nonthreatened and secure enough to share their innermost feelings. Health care professionals should reinforce the client's ability to make personal decisions and problem-solve. When appropriate, it is helpful to include family members in the problem-solving process.

It is important to identify situations that arouse feelings related to unmet needs. Discussions that stimulate recall of past experiences and positive outcomes and coping methods are beneficial. Assist individuals in manipulating their environment so that they can effect change. Recognize that helplessness may be a learned response and provide situations in which clients can exert some control over their environments.

In response to behavior that indicates hopelessness, do not become "Suzy Sunshine" and try to talk clients out of their depression. Instead, work with them to develop experiences that will provide them with positive feedback.

When working with depressed clients some additional considerations include the following:

Professionalism

- *Understand the disorder.* Health care professionals need to research and learn more about depressive disorders in order to help clients understand, cope, and seek professional help.

- *Listen to clients.* Health care professionals should encourage the client to discuss his or her feelings and listen in a nonjudgmental manner. If he or she cries, remember that tears can be therapeutic, and will help relieve the sadness. Say something like, "I understand how difficult this time is for you. Crying sometimes helps in dealing with a situation."

- *Encourage the client to seek professional help.*

- *Provide access to community resources.*

SUICIDE

Case Study: Suicide

Marlene has been angry for months but can't seem to express that anger to anyone. She is consumed with the anger and feels totally helpless. Panic sets in and Marlene makes a decision. She has decided that her life is no longer worth living. She is making elaborate plans to end it and has even set a date. She calls her sister, Marti, and makes a date to meet her for a cup of coffee. While they are having coffee, Marlene gives Marti a manila envelope with some personal belongings in it. When Marti opens it, Marlene comments, "It is just some things I want you to have if anything should happen to me."

Based on statistics collected by the National Center for Health Statistics of the Centers for Disease Control and Prevention (CDC) in 2012–2013, suicide was the 10th leading cause of death in the United States. The rate of suicide varies depending on age group, gender, ethnicity, and geographic location. In general, the highest rate is for older adults 85+ years of age. Many of these clients have visited their primary care provider just weeks prior to the suicide attempt. Middle-aged adults 45–64 years old also have a high rate of suicide. Young adults and seniors age 65–84 years old have a lower rate, and adolescents have a still lower rate.

The suicide rate for men is almost four times the rate for women; however, it is estimated that women attempt suicide three times as often as men. Among ethnic populations, Caucasians have the highest rate of suicide, followed closely by Native Americans, with African Americans and Asians having a rate about half the rate of Caucasians. Geography also has a significant effect on the suicide rate. Western states with a low population density have a significantly higher rate than more populous states. This may be because there is less opportunity for support. The leading reasons for suicide, in order of frequency, are relationships, health problems, job- or work-related problems (providers have one of the highest rates of suicides of any profession—mostly because they see so much death and despair), and financial difficulties. Other potential warning flags for suicide may include:

Cultural

- Major depression, other mental disorders, or substance use disorder
- Prior suicide attempts
- Exposure to suicide, mental disorders, or substance use disorders within the family

- Trauma or suicide of a friend, associate, or important person
- Being convicted of a serious crime
- Victim of family violence or sexual abuse

Four Stages of Contemplating Suicide

The individual contemplating suicide usually goes through the following four stages.

Stage #1

The individual's needs are not being met, so he or she becomes frustrated. Anger and hostility develop and the anger turns inward. Respond by trying to help the client identify unmet needs and the source of the frustration, and attempt to suggest means of meeting those needs.

Stage #2

Frustration leads to stress that becomes unbearable and panic sets in. The individual begins to look for a means of escape or to mobilize help. Be a resource to this client and carefully listen to his or her concerns. Try to move them back to Stage #1.

Stage #3

In an effort to seek help, the individual will communicate his or her helplessness to someone else. This is the point at which you can make a difference. Respond with care. Listen. Let the person know he or she is not alone. Keep in touch.

Stage #4

The individual then begins the suicide process. The person cannot help him- or herself. The feeling is that no one else cares, so "I'll end it all." The person begins to develop a plan to carry out the goal, then makes the preparations to carry out the plan. If under a provider's care for depression, the person may call to have a prescription refilled. Next, the person carries out the plan by taking the whole bottle of pills at one time. Intervention may be the only appropriate response at this stage.

Communicating Suicide Plans

Persons contemplating suicide often communicate their intentions before the attempt. The following are some signs that may indicate suicidal thoughts.

- Talk of killing themselves
- Talk of feeling they are in a hopeless situation

- Sudden change or withdrawal from normal social activities or interests
- Increased use of alcohol or drugs
- Excessive complaining about their responsibilities
- Extreme mood swings, possibly violent

Other approaches to communicating suicide plans may include one of the following coded message types. Coded messages are nonpersonal—it is something else that is dying. Just as verbal communication must be read in clusters, so these cues must be considered in the context of other messages.

- *Indirect*: "What would you do if I were not here to nag at you?"
- *Direct*: "I wonder what it feels like to die."
- *Coded verbal messages*: "I hate autumn—everything is dying."

Stop and Consider 8.3

Refer to "Case Study: Suicide" at the beginning of the section and respond to the following questions.

1. How does this case study fit with the four stages of contemplating suicide?

2. How does Marlene communicate her helplessness to her sister Marti?

Suicide Prevention

Suicide is a sign of extreme distress. It is not simply an attempt to obtain attention, nor is it a character flaw. It only indicates that the person has more pain than he or she feels capable of coping with. The best prevention for suicide is early recognition of the risk factors listed above and/or signals that the person is planning suicide. If you recognize that a person is contemplating suicide, do not leave him or her alone; call 911. Intervention is necessary immediately.

Risk factors can be reduced through psychotherapy or medical intervention. CBT attempts to train at-risk persons to consider alternative action when thoughts of suicide occur. Dialectical behavioral therapy (DBT) has been successful for persons with borderline personality disorder, characterized by mood instability, self-image problems, and mood swings. DBT attempts to help the person become aware of potentially suicidal feelings and instructs in the skills required to deal with them. A whole family of medications is available for the symptoms of depression and schizophrenia. Medications mask the symptoms but do not treat the disease. A major problem is failure of clients to faithfully take their medication, sometimes putting them at extreme risk.

The Therapeutic Response

Prevention is the only significant intervention. Remember, every threat or attempt of suicide is serious. This is a time to sit down, pull in close to the individual, and listen. Let the person know you really care, that you are a friend or professional, and that you will not leave or desert him or her. Tears are therapeutic, so cry if it is appropriate and you are sincere. Sometimes there is nothing you can do but sit in silence and perhaps hold the person's hand. Be empathetic, use both words and body language to convey feelings. 🎖 Allied health professionals often recognize the warning signs of suicide but are not skilled in techniques to handle suicidal clients on their own. Having a list of referrals on hand to provide to your client is suggested. Even calling to schedule the first appointment, with your client's permission, ensures a better outcome.

Professionalism

Paul Welter, in his book *How to Help a Friend* (1990), offers some therapeutic approaches (Welter, 1990):

- Listen, listen, listen.
- Do not give "pat answers" and easy advice.
- Make every effort to understand the mindset of the person.
- Communicate through the person's strong learning channel—visual, auditory, or touch/movement.
- Avoid arguments and power struggles. As a helper, you need to help the person to become less perturbed, not more perturbed. Direct the person away from a distasteful exchange.
- Let yourself feel some of the other person's suffering, and acknowledge the reality of his or her suffering. By responding in an empathic way, you may come across as saying, "I care." This is sometimes an effective way to reduce the amount of self-hatred.

It is helpful to let the person know that you see the pain and agony he or she is going through and that you care. Encourage the person to talk about how he or she is feeling and why. Ask what you can do to help, and be sincere in your offer.

Have a list of appropriate referrals. When in doubt as to your actions as a health care professional, ask your employer. Do not wait. Time is important in potential suicide situations. Call the toll-free National Suicide Prevention Lifeline at (800) 273-TALK (8255), available 24/7.

WHAT ABOUT THOSE LEFT BEHIND?

Suicide is a terribly wrong answer to whatever difficulties individuals may be facing. The suicide victim is gone, but family and friends live on suffering the consequences of suicide for the rest of their lives. Those left behind wonder what they could have done differently. They often blame themselves for the death of a family member or friend. Suicide shatters entire families and lingers on. These family members may suffer depression as a result of the death of a loved one. Physical problems, anxiety, divorce, and loss of income may also be experienced.

When one dies a natural death, usually empathy and compassion are expressed. Others want to comfort the one(s) left behind and rally in support. In the case of a suicide, family members may be treated differently (i.e., judged, condemned, and even blamed for the death). Suicide carries a stigma with it that those left behind must endure.

Suicide survivor support groups either online or in person are a great benefit for those left behind. Listen to survivors in a nonjudgmental way and encourage them to verbalize their feelings. Allow them to cry, and cry with them if it is appropriate. Be as supportive as possible.

Stop and Consider 8.4

News media often report stories in which individuals not only commit suicide, but take the lives of many other innocent victims as well. For example, an airline pilot who decides life is not worth living crashes into the side of a mountain, taking his life and the lives of the passengers. Or a train engineer who increases the train's speed, causing a derailment that kills himself and many passengers.

1. If you were a family member or a survivor left behind, how might you feel?

2. What would help you come to acceptance of such a tragedy?

3. What support groups might be helpful?

SUMMARY

Depressive disorders impact many people regardless of age, gender, race, ethnicity, or financial status. Depression is the leading cause of disability and can strike children, adolescents, adults, and older adults. Creating a nonthreatening environment in which clients can express their innermost feelings, knowing that they will not be belittled or made to feel inferior in any way, is important to the healing process. By being alert to danger signs, the health care professional can be a resource and provide support to depressed or suicidal clients. Listening carefully for any danger signs that the client may be suicidal is critical. An easy mnemonic can be used to remember the warning signs: IS PATH WARM?

I	Ideation		W	Withdrawal
S	Substance abuse		A	Anger
P	Purposelessness		R	Recklessness
A	Anxiety		M	Mood changes
T	Trapped			
H	Hopelessness			

Remember those left behind and provide support and encouragement to them. They must live with the consequences of suicide for the rest of their lives.

EXERCISES

Exercise 1

Identify your personal responses when feeling "blue" or "down in the dumps." Are these responses healthy or unhealthy? Do they promote resolution to problems or mask and internalize the problem? This exercise is designed for your use only and need not be shared with others.

Exercise 2

Using the Internet, look for self-help bulletin boards or other electronic reference sources that could help you, family members, or clients understand and manage depression. Make a list of the resources found to share with the class.

Exercise 3

Using the Internet, look for self-help bulletin boards or other electronic reference sources that could help you, family members, or clients understand suicide, those at risk, and intervention approaches. List each resource and summarize pertinent information contained in each site. Begin with the Centers for Disease Control and Prevention Web site (*www.cdc.gov*).

Exercise 4

Briefly describe how you would feel and how you would respond to the following situations. These exercises can be used in small group settings or can be completed independent of others.

1. Your client's medical record indicates that he has recently been diagnosed with persistent depressive disorder. He has been on antidepressants for 10 days now and tells you they are not working.

   I feel _____.

   I would say _____ .

2. Nancy Elwood bursts into tears as you ask about the reason for the visit today. She tells you her husband died 3 weeks ago of a massive heart attack. She says she can't sleep, is not eating well, feels listless, and has no interest in going on without him.

   I feel _____.

   I would say _____ .

3. Sonya brings her newborn in for his 6-week checkup. Little Danny seems to be just fine. When you ask how Sonya is doing, she tears up and says she is a wreck and hasn't shared this with anyone else because she is afraid she will be considered a bad mother and perhaps Danny would be taken out of her care.

   I feel _____.

   I would say _____ .

4. Your older client Willie Jenkins is being seen today because of a flare-up of gout. While taking his vitals he tells you he has been feeling depressed lately.

   I feel _____.

   I would say _____ .

5. Willie Jenkins is back for a complete physical examination today. He tells you he hates the fall season because everything is dying. He thinks he will die soon too.

   I feel _____.

   I would say _____ .

REVIEW QUESTIONS

Multiple Choice

1. Major depression is also known by what other name?
   a. Clinical depression
   b. Reactive depression
   c. Bipolar depression
   d. Persistent depressive disorder

2. Which statement applies to reactive depression?
   a. Comes from within
   b. Is considered the most temporary form of depression
   c. Is also known as PPND
   d. Is also known as seasonal pattern disorder

3. What is the treatment of choice for seasonal pattern disorder?
   a. Hospitalization
   b. Antidepressants
   c. Psychotherapy
   d. Light therapy

4. Which type of depression is also known as the baby blues?
   a. Persistent depressive depression
   b. Psychotic depression
   c. Peripartum-onset depression
   d. Reactive depression

5. Which type of depression alternates between extreme highs of mania and severe lows of hypomanic episodes?
   a. Psychotic depression
   b. Bipolar depression
   c. Seasonal pattern disorder
   d. Reactive depression

Short Answer

6. What is one of the two internationally recognized sets of diagnostic criteria references used to diagnose depression?

7. List five signs and symptoms of depression.

8. Which age group is at highest risk of suicide?

9. What is the term for actions such as making threats, spreading rumors, attacking someone physically or verbally, and excluding another intentionally from a group?

10. What is the method of treating disease, especially psychic disorders, by mental rather than pharmacological means?

FOR FURTHER CONSIDERATION

1. How would you respond therapeutically to the client experiencing reactive depression?

2. Discuss the impact of depression on each stage of the life cycle. How would you respond therapeutically to each age group?

3. Role-play a suicide scenario, with a classmate going through the four stages of contemplating suicide; use the mnemonic IS PATH WARM.

CASE STUDIES

Case Study 1

For months Esther, a travel agent, has felt very sad. She feels extremely fatigued and lethargic. She finds it difficult to sleep at night, and her appetite has decreased. Though reading was once a passion of hers, lately she lacks the concentration to even focus on the morning paper. She no longer enjoys activities with her friends and family. She is plagued with feelings of hopelessness; often she struggles to make it out of bed in the morning. She finds herself asking what the point is to her life, and wonders if life is even worth living.

1. Identify the symptoms of depression given in this scenario.

2. If you were Esther's friend, how would you respond therapeutically?

3. Does Esther need treatment for her depression?

Case Study 2

Timmy, a second-grader, wasn't feeling like himself. A month ago his best friend moved to another city, leaving Timmy feeling sad, miserable, and with no one to play with. His mom and dad were worried because he was no longer interested in kite-flying, something he had really enjoyed for a long time. Timmy also tried to make excuses for why he should stay home from school. Sometimes Timmy wouldn't go to sleep at night, and he wasn't interested in eating any of his favorite foods. His parents worried about how sad he always seemed. After a month of worry, his parents decided to take Timmy to a family counselor.

1. Is it possible a second-grader could be experiencing depression?

2. What symptoms did Timmy have that indicate depression?

3. How do you think the counselor will help Timmy?

REFERENCES AND RESOURCES

Please note that because Internet resources are of a time-sensitive nature and URL addresses may change or be deleted, searches should also be conducted by association and/or topic.

American Academy of Child and Adolescent Psychiatry. *Facts for families*. Retrieved from www.aacap.org.

American Foundation for Suicide Prevention. (2013). Facts and figures. In *Understanding Suicide*. Retrieved from https://www.afsp.org/understanding-suicide/facts-and-figures.

American Psychiatric Publishing. (2013). *Diagnostic and statistical manual of mental disorders* (5th ed.). Arlington, VA: Author.

Centers for Disease Control and Prevention. (2008). National Center for Injury Prevention and Control, Division of Violence Prevention. Suicide: data sources. In *Injury prevention and control: Division of Violence Prevention*. Retrieved from www.cdc.gov/violenceprevention/suicide/datasources.html.

Centers for Disease Control and Prevention. (2013). *The relationship between bullying and suicide: What we know and what it means for schools*. Retrieved from www.cdc.gov/violenceprevention/pdf/bullying-suicide-translation-final-a.pdf.

Centers for Disease Control and Prevention. (2015). *Suicide: Facts at a glance (2015)*. Retrieved March 29, 2015, from www.cdc.gov/violenceprevention/pdf/suicide-datasheet-a.pdf.

Centers for Medicare and Medicaid Services. (2010). *International classification of diseases, 10th Revision, Clinical Modification*. Washington, DC: Author.

Frisch, N. C., & Frisch, L. E. (2010). *Psychiatric mental health nursing* (4th ed.). Albany, NY: Thomson Delmar Learning.

Lindh, W. Q., Pooler, M. S., Tamparo C. D., & Dahl, B. M. (2014). *Comprehensive medical assisting: Administrative and clinical competencies* (5th ed.). Albany, NY: Thomson Delmar Learning.

Milliken, M. E., & Honeycutt. (2012). *Understanding human behavior: A guide for health care providers* (8th ed.). Albany, NY: Thomson Delmar Learning.

National Institute of Mental Health. (2015). Suicide in America: Frequently asked questions. Retrieved from www.nimh.nih.gov/health/publications/suicide-in-america/index.shtml.

Tamparo, C. D. (2016). *Diseases of the human body* (6th ed.). Philadelphia: F. A. Davis.

Chapter 9

The Therapeutic Response to Clients with Substance-Related and Addictive Disorders

CHAPTER OBJECTIVES

After completing this chapter, the learner should be able to:

- Define key terms as presented in the glossary.

- Compare substance dependence and substance abuse.

- Describe physiological and psychological dependence on a drug.

- List eight substances commonly abused and their effects on the human body.

- Identify the reasons clients often give for abusing their substance of choice.

- Describe important characteristics for addiction treatment.

- Discuss the therapeutic approach to clients with substance abuse and addictive disorders.

- Identify the role of family and friends with those who have substance-related and addictive disorders.

INTRODUCTION

Substance abuse and addiction, referred to as *substance use disorders* (*SUDs*), continue to be a major health and social problem in our society. SUDs gravely impact the general public, the demands on health care, family dynamics, and the individual. Addictions are serious and may cause chronic diseases that can be life-threatening.

DIAGNOSIS OF SUBSTANCE USE DISORDERS

Most clients *use* drugs of one kind or another for medical reasons and do so according to instructions. To *misuse* a drug implies that the directions for the drug use are exceeded. The *abuse* of a drug implies that it is used for other than medical purposes. Any drug can be used inappropriately. The lines between use, misuse, and abuse can be easily blurred, causing a problem. Individuals who are dependent on or abuse substances do so for many reasons, but generally there is a strong need to relieve tension, to relax, to forget about their troubles, and to help them cope with the daily demands of society.

Recreational drugs, taken for pleasure rather than for medical reasons, often lead to addiction and can cause health and social issues, depression and anxiety, crime, and death from an overdose. Most, but not all, recreational drugs are illegal. The *Diagnostic and Statistical Manual of Mental Disorders* (DSM-5), used by mental health care professionals to promote accurate diagnosis and treatment of mental disorders, combines the categories of substance abuse and substance dependence into a single disorder identified on a scale from mild to severe.

Substance Dependence

Substance dependence refers to substance use during a 12-month period that leads to significant impairment, manifested by *two* or more of the following: (1) tolerance defined as the need to take increased amounts of the substance to achieve the desired result and/or markedly diminished effect when using the same amount of the substance; (2) characteristic withdrawal for the substance or taking a closely related substance to relieve withdrawal; (3) taking the substance in larger amounts over a longer period than intended; (4) desire for the substance is persistent or efforts to control the substance use are unsuccessful; (5) major time is spent in activities to obtain the substance, use the substance, or recover from the effects of the substance; (6) social or occupational activities are diminished because of substance use; and (7) use of the substance continues in spite of persistent or recurrent physical or psychological problems associated with the substance.

Substance Abuse

Substance abuse refers to substance use during a 12-month period that leads to significant impairment manifested by *one* or more of the following: (1) recurrent substance use that results in a failure to fulfill major obligations at work, school, or home; (2) continued use of the substance in situations that are physically hazardous to self and others; (3) recurrent substance-related legal problems; and (4) continued use of the substance in spite of persistent or recurrent physical or psychological problems associated with the substance.

Addiction

Addiction is defined as either physiological or psychological dependence on a substance that is beyond voluntary control. *Physiological* or *physical dependence* implies that the body chemistry has been so affected that withdrawal from the substance produces a physical reaction at the cellular level, sometimes with severe complications. *Psychological dependence* means that the individual craves the substance being abused for the "good feeling" it provides. This need for the substance and the support it gives is viewed as a coping mechanism.

There still is debate among professionals as to whether addiction is a disease, is a choice, has a genetic and/or developmental basis, or is a combination of all three. It is not the purpose of this text to bring an end to this debate. The DSM-5, however, classifies addiction as a disease. While it is likely true that an at-risk individual for addiction makes a conscious choice at one point to smoke, drink, or use a drug, current evidence supports the disease factor and/or a genetic/developmental factor in substance-related and addictive disorders. Accepting drug dependence or abuse as a disease, however, does not totally erase or excuse the responsibility of an individual with an addictive disorder.

A well-known program that shows success with addicted people is Alcoholics Anonymous (AA). AA is a self-help organization for alcohol and substance abusers that is self-supporting and nondenominational. Narcotics Anonymous (NA), an offshoot of AA, closely follows the AA program but specifically ministers to those addicted to narcotics. The AA and NA programs are based on following a 12-step program that helps individuals live without their drug of choice. AA and NA sponsor meetings in nearly every community in the country to help people with addictions develop a close bond with others with similar problems (Figure 9-1). AA/NA believes that people with addictive disorder are completely responsible for their own recovery. There is a strong religious flavor to both AA and NA that some individuals dislike; however, statistics indicate that people following a 12-step program and who are active in AA/NA meetings have a 50% greater chance at success in recovery.

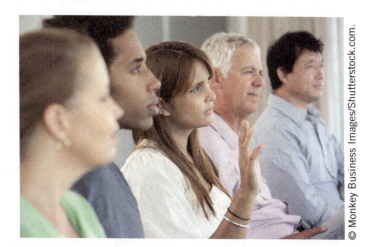

FIGURE 9-1   A meeting at a support group.

COMMONLY ABUSED SUBSTANCES

Some of the more commonly abused substances are identified here, with just a brief overview of their use and effect.

Nicotine is highly addictive in any form. Nicotine or tobacco is smoked or chewed. Even when many cities are banning smoking from all public places, smoking is still seen as a socially acceptable form of addiction. However, some health care professionals label nicotine addiction as a slow form of suicide. It is a chronic and relapsing addiction that often results in serious illness. Smokers have a risk of cancers of the lungs, mouth, throat, stomach, and bladder, and are prone to cardiovascular disease. The danger of second-hand smoke is also well known. The Centers for Disease Control and Prevention (CDC) states that tobacco is the single greatest cause of preventable death in the United States. Because nicotine is physiologically addictive, the smoker who quits experiences physical withdrawal symptoms that may include anxiety, agitation, weight gain, and insomnia. It is very difficult to stop using nicotine. Many who are addicted are unable to do so without assistance. Support groups may be helpful; also, there are drugs available to make breaking the addiction and preventing relapse more manageable. They come in the form of prescription gum, patches, and oral medications.

Alcohol, both socially acceptable and legal, is also one of the most commonly abused drugs in society. Alcohol produces a temporary feeling of well-being, but is a depressant that acts upon the central nervous system. Intoxication depends on the amount of alcohol in the bloodstream, with an amount between 0.08 and 0.10 being considered as legally intoxicated. An intoxicated person suffers slowed thinking and reaction time, impaired vision, poor coordination, and altered judgment as a result of the drug's action. After the initial euphoria and increased motor activity come clumsiness and staggering gait. Nausea and vomiting may occur. Withdrawal symptoms include anxiety, insomnia, tremors, and delirium. Alcoholism is generally identified in three stages: early-, middle-, and late-stage alcoholism.

In the early stage, the occasional drinker begins to drink to avoid problems or to bolster confidence. There is an increase in the individual's ability to tolerate alcohol, and large amounts may be consumed without the individual appearing impaired. In the middle stage, drinking is more intense and begins earlier in the day. The individual is losing control over drinking, usually denies a problem with alcohol, may have blackouts, and begins to suffer serious physical symptoms. In the late stage of alcoholism, the individual is totally obsessed with alcohol, internal organs have been damaged, malnutrition is evident, and death follows if treatment is not received.

Over-the-Counter and Prescription Medications

Cough/cold medicines are readily available, usually in syrup or capsule form to be swallowed. When abused, they can cause euphoria, slurred speech, increased heart rate and blood pressure, numbness, dizziness, confusion, paranoia, altered visual perceptions, and increased acid in body fluids. On the street, they are referred to as Robotripping, Robo, and Triple C. The commercial names are varied, but usually include the initials "DM." Many of these medications are available only from behind the counter at the pharmacy rather than off the shelf.

Prescription medications commonly abused include opioids, sedatives, stimulants, and anabolic steroids. Throughout the next section, refer to Table 9-1 for the Drug Enforcement Agency's list of controlled substances.

Opioids are used medically to control pain. They also can be used to reduce gastrointestinal motility, to curb nausea and vomiting, and to suppress the cough reflex. They can cause drowsiness, constipation, euphoria, confusion, slowed breathing, even death. Opioids come from the opium poppy seed, but are also synthetically made in a laboratory. Hydrocodone, oxycodone, morphine, and codeine are examples of opiates. When abused, stupor, decreased respiration, unconsciousness, and coma can result. Opioids are listed in all five of the Drug Schedule classifications, and are highly addictive when abused. These drugs are generally injected, swallowed, smoked, or snorted. Withdrawal symptoms include watery eyes, runny nose, decreased appetite, irritability, tremors, chills and sweats, cramps, and nausea.

Sedatives include tranquilizers and depressants and are commonly swallowed or injected. They depress the central nervous system, causing symptoms of lethargy and sleepiness. Speech may be slurred, heart rate is slowed, and blood pressure may be lowered. These drugs have significant use therapeutically, but can be highly addictive, leading to both physiological and psychological dependence. Sedatives are often prescribed for the treatment of certain stress disorders, for relief of insomnia and pain, and to prevent seizures. Dependence on these drugs may be so strong that individuals cannot function normally after withdrawal. Valium is one of the most abused drugs in this category. Withdrawal symptoms may not occur until a week or more after discontinuing the drug and may include anxiety, insomnia, and tremors.

Stimulants increase alertness, attention, energy, blood pressure, heart rate, and respiration. They include amphetamines such as Adderall that is often prescribed to treat those diagnosed with attention-deficit/hyperactivity

Legal

TABLE 9-1   The Drug Enforcement Agency's List of Controlled Substances

SCHEDULE I

- Substance has high potential for abuse.

- No currently accepted medical use in treatment.

- Lack of safety for use of the substance under medical supervision.

Examples include marijuana*, heroin, Ecstasy, psilocybin, LSD, peyote, synthetic cathyinones, hallusinogens, DHB.

* The **Drug Enforcement Agency (DEA)** has asked the **Food and Drug Administration (FDA)** to reclassify marijuana to Schedule II in light of recent states' legislation making recreational marijuana legal.

SCHEDULE II

- Substance has high potential for abuse.

- Has a currently accepted medical use or medical use accepted with severe restrictions.

- Abuse may lead to severe psychological or physical dependence.

Examples include cocaine, Ritalin, opium, oxycodone, morphine, amphetamines, secobarbital.

SCHEDULE III

- Substance has less potential for abuse than substances in Schedules I and II.

- Substance has a currently accepted medical use.

- Abuse may lead to moderate or low physical dependence or high psychological dependence.

Examples include anabolic steroids, ketamine, paregoric, hydrocodone, Rohypnol.

SCHEDULE IV

- Substance has a low potential for abuse relative to substances in Schedule III.

- Substance has a currently accepted medical use.

- Abuse may lead to limited physical dependence or psychological dependence relative to substances in Schedule III.

Examples include Valium, Librium, Xanax, Ambien, Darvon.

SCHEDULE V

- Substance has low potential for abuse relative to substances in Schedule IV.

- Substance has a currently accepted medical use.

- Abuse may lead to limited physical dependence or psychological dependence relative to substances in Schedule IV.

Examples include cough suppressants containing small amounts of codeine and preparations containing small amounts of opium.

While the federal law has five schedules, some states have added a Schedule VI to cover substances abused recreationally. They include substances such as those found in spray paints, and nitrous oxide, found in many types of aerosol cans. Because pseudoephedrine is widely used in the manufacture of methamphetamine, some states have strict regulations regarding the sale of any cold remedy containing pseudoephedrine. These drugs include Sudafed and Actifed.

Adapted from United States Code of Federal Regulations, Title 21, Chapter 13.

disorder or ADHD. When abused, they can cause dangerously high body temperature, irregular heartbeat, seizures, and heart failure. They can be swallowed, snorted, smoked, or injected.

Anabolic steroids are made to be used for conditions caused by low levels of steroid hormones in the body. They are often abused to enhance athletic or sexual performance and physical appearance. They come in many forms—tablets, capsules, liquids, gels and creams, patches, or injectable solutions. Abuse can result in fluid retention, yellowing of the skin, kidney and liver damage, high blood pressure, or changes in cholesterol leading to stroke or heart attack. Behavioral changes include aggression, extreme mood swings, paranoia, delusions, and irritability.

Recreational Drugs

Bath salts (synthetic cathyinones) are a family of stimulant drugs that are likely swallowed, snorted, or injected. Many have been banned by the DEA. Some of the street names are Bloom, Cloud Nine, Cosmic Blast, Ivory, Vanilla Sky, and White Lightning. They cause increased heart rate and blood pressure, euphoria, increased sex drive, paranoia, agitation, and hallucinations. Over time, there is a breakdown of skeletal muscle tissue and kidney failure.

Cocaine comes from the coca plant, but can also be manufactured in a laboratory. Cocaine is a strong stimulant to the central nervous system, and is used medically as an anesthetic. In surgery, it can deaden a local area and produce vasoconstriction to reduce bleeding at the site. When abused, cocaine is sniffed or snorted into the nose, rubbed on the mucous membranes, or injected. It creates a euphoria that lasts about 30 minutes, leaving an individual with a greater need each time to have more. It is quick and severe in its addiction and creates multiple side effects that can include cardiac arrhythmias, seizures, respiratory arrest, and death. Crack cocaine is smoked. Withdrawal symptoms include apathy, long periods of sleep, irritability, and depression.

DHB (Rohypnol and gamma hydroxybutyrate) are two of the most common substances present when drug-facilitated sexual assaults occur. GHB is usually taken orally. It comes in a powder that easily dissolves in liquids. It is clear, odorless, tasteless, and nearly undetectable in a drink. Side effects are nausea, delusions, vertigo, hallucinations, respiratory distress, loss of consciousness, slowed heart rate, and coma. The use of this "date rape" drug makes it easier for the offender to render the victim physically incapacitated or helpless and unable to consent to sexual activity.

Hallucinogens excite the central nervous system. They have no medical use. These drugs cause hallucinations, mood changes, and delusions. They elevate all vital signs and are highly addicting. Abusers may experience the hallucinations for up to a year following treatment and withdrawal. Most abusers lose touch with reality. They also may injure themselves or others while under the influence. Paranoia, psychosis, and unpleasant "flashbacks" are common. These drugs are usually in the form of lysergic acid diethylamide (LSD), ketamine, mescaline (peyote), and psilocybin (magic mushroom).

Heroin, an opioid from morphine, comes from the opium poppy plant. It depresses the central nervous system and affects the brain's pleasure systems, making it difficult for the brain to perceive pain. It is often cut with nutmeg, sucrose, starch, flour, or talcum powder. It is known as Horse, Smack, Dope, Mud, or Dog. There is an immediate euphoric surge or rush upon use. There is diminished mental capacity and decreased respiration that can lead to respiratory failure. It is commonly injected, snorted, or smoked. Withdrawal involves severe cramps, muscle spasms, and pain.

Inhalants—unstable and unpredictable chemical substances in such household items as glue, gasoline, paint thinners, and aerosol spray paints are often abused by teenagers seeking a "cheap" thrill. They can produce significant behavioral and psychological changes in an individual, such as apathy or aggression and dizziness or slurred speech. On the street, they are known as Poppers, Snappers, and Laughing Gas. The use of inhalants is widespread and dangerous, but often is not classified as addictive because only a small portion of users become dependent. However, abuse of inhalants can lead to coma or, in some cases, even death.

Marijuana (Cannabis) is a drug under much debate as more states move to make it legal. It is believed beneficial in reducing nausea and vomiting for those receiving chemotherapy. It is effective in the treatment of certain types of seizures. Marijuana is, however, recognized by the DEA (see Table 9-1) as a Schedule I drug with little or no benefit and high potential for abuse. (Refer to the note in Table 9-1 regarding marijuana.) Marijuana comes from the dried tops of the cannabis or hemp plant. It has many different street names, including grass, pot, weed, and joint. It is smoked or swallowed. A state of euphoria, altered judgment, and altered perception results from its use. Slowed thinking and reaction time, as well as confusion and impaired balance, are exhibited. A person abusing marijuana may have symptoms of lethargy, hunger, agitation, cough, and frequent respiratory infections. There is a debate among experts as to whether there are withdrawal symptoms from the use of marijuana.

Amphetamines excite the central nervous system. Used medically, it can treat short-term fatigue, some respiratory conditions, depression, and narcolepsy. *Methamphetamine* is the most commonly abused drug in this category. It is easily manufactured by anyone having the right ingredients, and is a major concern for law enforcement officials around the country. The street names are Crank, Chalk, Crystal, Fire, Ice, Meth, and Speed. Methamphetamine gives the user a short-term feeling of exhilaration, energy, and increased mental alertness. Adverse effects include aggression, violence, psychotic behavior, paranoia, hallucinations, cardiac and neurological damage, and impaired memory and learning. Withdrawal symptoms are the same as for cocaine.

OTHER ADDICTIONS

Health care professionals may become aware of other addictions that can occur in clients' lives. Individuals may become addicted to sexual activity, to gambling, to shopping, to spending hours on the Internet, or to any activity that gives a high-adrenaline rush to the pleasure center of their brains. Some authorities believe compulsive overeating may constitute an addiction to food. As food becomes more palatable, more pleasurable, and more refined, it also is consumed in much larger quantities than necessary. When food becomes an addiction, it is being consumed not to satisfy a normal hunger, but to achieve a pleasurable reward and the belief that "I am worthy and loved." no matter what the consequences.

TREATMENT

Primary care professionals who are alert and diligent about getting a thorough social history from clients may uncover a tendency on the part of clients to drink too much or to rely on drugs to cope with daily living. Because many health problems are associated with substance dependence and abuse, health care professionals may be the first to diagnose a substance dependence or abuse problem (Figure 9-2).

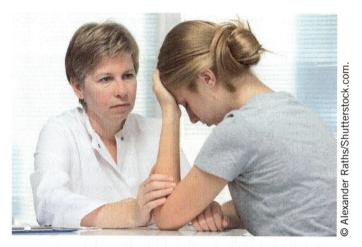

FIGURE 9-2   A young woman discusses substance abuse concerns with a health care professional.

Stop and Consider 9.2

You are a medical assistant interviewing Jana, the expectant mother identified in the opening case study. You are asking her the questions on the social history form. She tells you she does not smoke. She does not drink coffee, but she drinks cola products nearly every day. In response to the questions on alcohol, she is a little evasive. Since Jana volunteered to you earlier that she is fearful she might be an alcoholic, you know the goal is for her to be truthful to you now.

1. What might you say to open the communication?

2. What questions will you ask?

Mental health care professionals working in concert with primary care professionals also often reveal substance dependence and/or abuse. The first step is to recognize the problem and the second step is proper treatment. Most treatment plans will include a number of days of **detoxification** as an inpatient in a treatment facility, to begin to rid the body of the abused substance. This period may include the administration of medications. Following detoxification, treatment must continue with close and careful monitoring, counseling, and support to enable individuals to remain free of substance abuse. Studies show the following factors are significant in the worsening health of individuals addicted to a substance: female gender, living alone, problem use of opioids and/or alcohol, having no medical insurance, older age, and clients who abuse more than one substance. When the brain has been affected by the abuse of substances, many individuals turn to risky sexual behaviors, thus increasing their health risk for transmission of infectious diseases, including HIV.

A client needing treatment feels caught in a vicious cycle that begins with excessive use of a drug: disapproval–self-recrimination–guilt–rationalization and denial (defense mechanisms)–continued excessive use of a drug (see Figure 9-3). One of the keys to successful treatment is to break this cycle so the client can move toward recovery. Appropriate treatment will likely be different for each client, but the following points are important:

- No single treatment will work for everyone.
- Treatment should be readily available, even without medical insurance; unfortunately, that is not the reality in today's world.
- Medical detoxification is only the beginning of treatment for long-term drug use.
- An adequate period of time is necessary for treatment effectiveness.
- Individual and/or group counseling is critical to treatment.
- Treatment should tend to *all* the needs of the individual, including medical services, family therapy, vocational rehabilitation, and social and legal services as necessary.
- Certain medications are increasingly successful in assisting the treatment process.
- Treatment for addictive disorders is a long-term process and often requires multiple episodes of treatment.

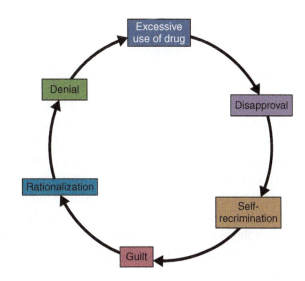

FIGURE 9-3   Cycle of drug dependency.

The Role of Family and Friends in Substance-Related and Addictive Disorders

It is important to briefly discuss the role of family members and friends in the treatment of substance-related and addictive disorders. The disease is a problem that affects the entire family. Everyone near the addict suffers. It is not possible or beneficial to try to cajole, beg, or intimidate the person to change. Persons with substance use disorders can only decide for themselves to give up the drugs they abuse. Family members may even become part of the problem when they try to conceal their loved one's addiction. This is done by making excuses to employers, giving money when they should not, and generally enabling the drug-dependent person to remain dependent, thereby not facing up to the reality of the problem. There are many support groups dealing with the problem of codependency and numerous books written on the subject. Health professionals must also be careful not to become codependent to the problem.

Self-Awareness

There are five Cs to recall when working with substance-dependent clients. They were identified many years ago, and have been useful to many who live or work with drug dependency. Remember:

- I did not CAUSE the disease.
- I cannot CURE the disease.
- I cannot CONTROL the disease or the substance-dependent client.
- And if I try to, I CONTRIBUTE to the problem,
- And I go CRAZY.

The Therapeutic Response

Professionalism

Health care professionals may have more difficulty maintaining a therapeutic relationship with addicted clients than with clients seeking other kinds of medical care because the chance for relapse is so great. It can be depressing to watch a client slip back into destructive habits after many months, even years of being free from the abuse. Health care professionals must strive for an unbiased approach to their clients and see their role as one of helping clients choose recovery. Collaboration will be expected from all professionals caring for the person with an addiction problem. The following points can help health care professionals be more therapeutic in their approach:

- Become educated regarding substance-related and addictive disorders. You cannot be therapeutic toward individuals with a problem you do not understand.

- Be alert to people at risk in your client population. These can include, but are not limited to, children of drug dependents, people with high-stress lives, individuals who have easy access to substances, individuals with unresolved emotional problems, and individuals with chronic and debilitating health issues.

- Encourage clients to seek treatment when there is a problem. Help them understand the available resources and make referrals as appropriate.

- Do not moralize or scold clients for their behavior. Everyone else does that to them.

- Manage any negative feelings you have.

- Do not be discouraged, and do not believe you can "fix it."

- Elicit the cooperation and participation of family members and friends in the treatment process. Help them understand the codependency cycle.

- Be tolerant of clients who relapse. Be willing to start again with clients who fail or drop out of treatment.

- Attitudes of compassion, understanding, patience, and acceptance are the best therapeutic approaches to drug-dependent clients. Such a relationship fosters positive motivation for the client who needs strong support in his or her recovery process.

SUMMARY

It is rare today to find a family that is not touched in one way or another by the problem of substance-related and addictive disorders. It is a major problem for society as a whole, as well as for all of health care. Health care professionals will be able to respond more therapeutically if they are well informed and are up to date on the latest developments for substance dependence and abuse. It is important to understand the culture of the community in which you are employed, to be nonjudgmental in your approach to drug-dependent clients, and to provide as much support as possible. Have a ready list of available resources and services for clients and their families. Here is a partial list of national resources:

- Alcoholics Anonymous: www.aa.org
- Narcotics Anonymous: www.na.org

- Drug Abuse Resistance Education: www.dare.com
- MedlinePlus (Substance Abuse Problems/Topics): www.nlm.nih.gov/medlineplus/substanceabuseproblems.html
- National Institute on Drug Abuse: www.nida.nih.gov
- Substance Abuse and Mental Health Services Administration (SAMHSA): www.samhsa.gov

EXERCISES

Exercise 1

If you live in an area large enough to have a treatment center for individuals who abuse drugs, interview the administrator or a counselor. If you are in an area that does not have any treatment facilities, search the Internet for treatment centers. Your goals are to discover the following:

1. What resources are available in the community?

2. What are the most commonly abused substances they see in their clients?

3. What factors make their treatment successful?

4. What problems are faced by clients when discharged?

5. What is the cost of treatment, and who pays if there is no health insurance?

6. How are families involved, if they are at all, in the treatment plan?

Write a summary of the information you received and describe what you learned from the experience.

Exercise 2

Using the Internet, research Alcoholics Anonymous to determine their 12-step program approach. Would these 12 steps work for individuals from all cultures? Justify your response.

Exercise 3

1. An Arab student in your nursing class says to you, "I'm not sure I can do the rehab rotation. Drugs and alcohol are forbidden in my culture. What do I say to my instructor?"

   You feel _____.

   You respond _____.

2. A friend says to you, "I sure like to party, and sometimes it is so good, I can't remember how I got home."

   You feel _____.

   You respond _____.

3. A client says to you, "My pain medication is no longer working so good. Can you make sure I get something stronger from the doc?"

   You feel _____.

   You respond _____.

4. A veteran from the war in Afghanistan comes to your clinic for his second round of drug addiction treatment.

   You feel _____.

   You respond _____.

Exercise 4

Write a brief paragraph about someone you know who abuses a substance. What is your response to that individual? Are you codependent? Why or why not? Describe any action you might be able to take to help that individual.

REVIEW QUESTIONS

Multiple Choice

1. What is the most commonly abused substance in the United States?

   a. Alcohol

   b. Prescriptive drugs

   c. Nicotine

   d. Methamphetamine

2. What is the standard tool used by mental health care professionals to promote accurate diagnosis and treatment of mental disorders called?

   a. ICD-10-CM   **c.** CPT

   b. SUD   **d.** DSM-5

3. What is the term for when the body chemistry is so affected that withdrawal from the substance produces a reaction at the cellular level?

   a. Physiological dependence   **c.** Chemical dependence

   b. Psychological dependence   **d.** Chemical abuse

4. What is the drug that may be abused, is currently listed as a Schedule I drug, but is now legal in a number of states?

   a. Cocaine   **c.** Valium

   b. Marijuana   **d.** Heroin

5. What classification of drugs excite the CNS; cause delusions, mood changes, and flashbacks; and are highly addictive?

   a. Inhalants   **c.** Stimulants

   b. Opioids   **d.** Hallucinogens

FOR FURTHER CONSIDERATION

1. You have just heard your 16-year-old daughter return home from a date. She is getting ready for bed. You step into her room to ask her how the date was and to kiss her good night. You are immediately overwhelmed by the smell of alcohol. What do you say? What will you do? Where might you go for resources?

2. The school board in your community has voted to randomly test for drugs all students who participate in extracurricular activities. Your son, a better-than-average football player, says he'll not play another day on the team if he has to pee in a cup for anyone. What is your response? Can you identify both positive and negative aspects of the school board's decision?

CASE STUDIES

Case Study 1

Your provider has asked you to put together some information for Jana, the client identified at the beginning of this chapter who is pregnant with her first child and believes she has an alcohol problem. What information will you include? What resources will you recommend to her? Identify any community resources available. Provide information about her health needs and the health needs of her unborn infant during pregnancy.

Case Study 2

Roxann Piersen is a long-term client in your ambulatory care medical center who suffers from severe headaches and debilitating back pain. You have reason to believe she is abusing her pain medications. Your chart notes indicate that either she or her pharmacy calls for refills on her prescription prior to the time when she should be out of her medications. You have two notes, one indicating she accidentally spilled most of her pills down the sink, and another note saying she lost the medications while on vacation. What action do you take? Explain.

REFERENCES AND RESOURCES

American Psychiatric Association. (2014). *Diagnostic and statistical manual of mental disorders* (5th ed.). Arlington, VA: American Psychiatric Association.

National Institute on Drug Abuse. www.nida.nih.gov.

Substance Abuse and Mental Health Services Administration (SAMHSA). www.samhsa.gov.

Tamparo, C. D. (2016). *Diseases of the human body* (6th ed.). Philadelphia: F. A. Davis.

Chapter 10

The Therapeutic Response to Clients with Life-Altering Illness

CHAPTER OBJECTIVES

After completing this chapter, the learner should be able to:

- Define key terms as presented in the glossary.
- Contrast acute illness, chronic illness, and life-altering illness.
- Identify typical phases of life-altering illness clients may experience.
- Describe several psychological effects of illness.
- Discuss the use of medications and life-altering illness.
- Discuss cultural influences on life-altering illness.
- Identify appropriate therapeutic responses to chronic and life-altering illness.

Opening Case Study

I was 25 years of age, and my daughter was just 7 months old, when I learned that a tumor on the right lobe of my thyroid gland had to be removed. Surgical procedures went well, and the surgeon felt everything would be all right. Four days later my surgeon came to the hospital room and asked if I would walk down to the sunroom with him. We sat down; he pulled his chair close to mine and took hold of my hand. "Billie, there is no easy way to tell you this, but your lab results came back positive for cancer. We must do radical surgery to remove the remainder of the thyroid and to see how far the cancer has spread." As his words began to sink in, he added, "I want you to call your husband. When he arrives, I will come back in to speak with him, too."

The next few days were rather a blur. The surgery was scheduled. Arrangements were made with a friend to take care of my daughter. My sister would come from Texas to help after surgery. At that time, the only treatment for cancer of this type was radical surgery. Because the surgeon was not sure if or how far the cancer might have metastasized, and the thoracic region has an abundance of lymph nodes, the surgery would be extensive. An incision was made from my right ear along the jaw line to the center of my chin. Another incision was made down the side of my neck and to my midthoracic region. A third incision was made around the front of my neck and out to the end of my right shoulder. I think of it now as being like a side of beef hung out to cure before being cut into serving portions. Or as my friend said, like a "live autopsy."

For three days after surgery I was kept heavily sedated. When I was lucid, the surgeon told me that he took two of my parathyroid glands as well as the thyroid. He told me I would need to take medicine the rest of my life—but he had saved my life. I was grateful. I also did not fully understand what would happen next. When I came home, I could not climb the few stairs to the bedroom, so I slept on the couch. The pain was so bad that I could not stand to have anything touch me; I could not even wear my clothes. My sister touched me lightly with a cotton ball, and I screamed with pain. I awoke one night with my body on fire. I could see a fire in the fireplace and I screamed for my husband. "I am on fire!" He said, "No, you're not." But I could feel my skin burning; I just couldn't smell the burned flesh. When I called the surgeon the next morning, his response was "Thank God. That burning sensation means your nerves are regenerating." (Too bad he hadn't told me to expect this.)

(continues)

231

Opening Case Study   (*Continued*)

For one entire year, I could not function without assistance. My sister stayed with me 6 weeks after the surgery, then friends and neighbors helped as much as possible. It was next to impossible to raise my right arm, to wash or comb my hair; even to dress myself was a chore. I could not pick up my daughter. She had to be put on my lap for me to hold and love. During this time, I learned that my other two parathyroid glands had atrophied from the trauma of surgery and were no longer functioning. Now I had no thyroid gland to secrete the thyroid hormones tetraiodothyronine (thyroxine or T4) and triiodothyronine (T3)—the hormones essential for life and that have many effects on body metabolism, growth, and development. I also had no parathyroid glands to secrete parathyroid hormone (PTH) necessary to regulate the amount of calcium in my blood. Calcium is a critical element for the nervous system, the muscular system, and the skeletal system. When calcium levels drop below normal (which mine certainly had by now), tingling sensations in the fingers and/or cramps in the muscles of the hands are common. The muscle cramps spread to all muscles, including the heart, which can be life-threatening.

Gradually, my life began to normalize. I was able to take care of myself, be the kind of mother I wanted to be, and go on with my life. Five years after surgery, our son was born. The surgeon had warned us that to have a child any earlier could be dangerous because of the increased hormone activity during pregnancy. I now thought I was home free; however, I still panicked each year when it was time for my annual physical examination. Would the cancer return?

Living with thyroid replacement medication is not too difficult, and keeping the replacement hormone at just the right level has been fairly simple. Regulating the calcium level in the blood is quite a different story. I faithfully took the medicine, including vitamin D. Most people do not require extra doses of Vitamin D because so many of our foods are fortified with it today.

After 20 years on this regime, I began to lose my appetite and then became extremely nauseous. The nausea became so severe I could not keep water or even ice chips down. I lost 20 pounds. My provider did not know what was happening, and I felt like he thought I was just making up my symptoms. When I got no relief, and began to run a fever because I was so dehydrated, I called the provider again. I told him I was on my way to the emergency room. If he wanted to meet me there, it was okay; otherwise I was going to seek out another provider. My provider met me at the emergency room and immediately called for an internist to review my case. Blood tests were run, and both my calcium levels and blood pressure were sky-high. Because vitamin D is stored in the body (primarily in the kidneys), taking large doses over a period of time can cause hypervitaminosis D (poisoning) and even death; my body had reached a dangerously high level. I spent a week in the hospital being pumped with IV fluids to flush out my system. It was discovered that some permanent damage had taken place in my kidneys.

I am still learning to live with this life-altering illness. A new calcium hormone has eliminated the need to take vitamin D now and my calcium level is fairly normal and stable. I have iatrogenic Horner's syndrome, causing problems with my right pupil dilating, ptosis of the right eyelid, and loss of sweating over the right side of my face. When I am overheated, half my face is white and dry while the other half is beet-red and sweaty.

I live a rich and full life in spite of these problems. I went back to school, earned my medical assisting degree, became certified, worked in a medical clinic, and later became the medical assisting program director at my alma mater. I rewrote the medical assisting curriculum into self-paced modules with open enrollment, in order to offer all students an equal opportunity for education. I am a coauthor of this text and of a major medical assistant text. I am about the best grandma around, and I am the first-mate on our 34-foot sailboat. We travel and have seen beautiful places around the world.

I decided long ago that my attitude was critical to my well-being. I accepted my life-altering illness. I choose to live life to the fullest in spite of it. I maintain a positive attitude, look for the good in everyone and everything, and encourage others. I am more sympathetic to individuals who have health issues because of my life experience. My hope is that everyone might experience health care professionals who listen, respect their clients, provide honest feedback, and genuinely care about the uniqueness of each person.

—Billie Lindh

Stop and Consider 10.1

After reading the opening case study, please respond to the following questions.

1. Do you think Billie's positive attitude has any impact on the way she lives her life with a life-altering illness?

2. Can you explain why she might be more sympathetic to individuals who have health issues in general?

3. How can advancements in medical and pharmaceutical technology provide hope for persons with life-altering illnesses?

INTRODUCTION

It can be very frightening when you or a loved one is given a serious diagnosis. Life-altering conditions can happen at any time and at any age. Questions flood our mind. Is there a cure for this disease/disorder? How will this impact my life? What changes will need to be made to cope with this diagnosis? How will this impact my finances? Most of us have no training or experience with life-altering illnesses. Good health is often taken for granted. As illness progresses from a minor inconvenience to a life-altering circumstance, meeting the client's needs as well as those of the family in a therapeutic manner becomes increasingly challenging.

ILLNESS TYPES

Most illnesses are unexpected and always bring daily and/or life changes. Illnesses come in many different forms, some lasting only hours and others impacting lives in significant ways for months or years. Illnesses can be characterized as **acute**, **chronic**, and **life-altering**.

Acute Illness

Clients with acute illness experience a rapid onset of the illness with severe symptoms, most often for a short duration. These clients may not be able to perform the tasks of daily living and may be unable to continue their occupational employment until the illness has run its course. Acute illnesses can be classified as an inconvenience, and do not normally result in life changes. Examples of acute illnesses include a cold, the flu, tonsillitis, or rashes. Left untreated, however, acute illnesses may progress into chronic conditions. Symptoms of acute illnesses may include fever, diarrhea, nausea, vomiting, stomach cramps, and inflammation. Medical personnel need to help the client understand any implications of the diagnosis and assist them in making decisions regarding their medical care. For example, serious back strain can lead to temporary loss of work, medication treatment, physical therapy, or even lifestyle change when employment requires heavy lifting.

Professional

Chronic Illness

An illness is usually labeled chronic when its symptoms linger over a period of time, showing little change or decreased progression. While some chronic illnesses may be cured within a few weeks or months, many may become life-altering, lasting a lifetime. **Curative care** is provided for those conditions that have a possibility of a cure. Chronic illnesses typically have a significant impact on clients, necessitating life-altering changes as they attempt to cope with the illness, comply with treatments, and deal with possible side effects. The illness may gradually debilitate and shorten their life span. At this point, **palliative care** or even **hospice care** (see Chapter 11) may be required. Palliative care relieves or alleviates symptoms without curing while hospice care provides a program of palliative care and supportive services. This care may be provided in the home or in a hospice center.

It is not the purpose of this text to identify specific diseases and clients' possible reactions to them, but the following are examples of chronic illnesses that may become life-altering.

- Arthritis
- Fibromyalgia
- Multiple sclerosis
- Type I diabetes mellitus
- Diabetic neuropathy
- Cancer
- Acquired immunodeficiency syndrome (AIDS)
- Human immunodeficiency virus (HIV)
- Chronic obstructive pulmonary disease (COPD)
- Alzheimer's disease
- Stroke
- Parkinson's disease

Life-Altering Illness

Case Study: Life-Altering Illness

Kyle has been an active 17-year-old enjoying success on the basketball team his senior year. Recently, Kyle has been complaining of headaches and is having trouble with speech and coordination. After several tests have been run, Kyle and his family are given the diagnosis of a brain tumor. Several treatment plans are discussed and a prognosis given.

A life-altering illness can be defined as an illness that affects or limits the quality of life of an individual. Some chronic illnesses and most life-threatening illnesses are life-altering illnesses. When chronic illness progresses to the stage when death is the inevitable result, the illness is defined as *life-threatening*; however, some chronic illnesses and most life-threatening illnesses are categorized as life-altering illnesses. A life-altering diagnosis creates feelings of powerlessness and lack of control. Hope should always be maintained, however, as in some cases the disease may be fought for years before ultimately ending in death. Therapeutic responses should emphasize a positive outlook (Figure 10-1).

There is a fine line between a life-altering illness and a life-threatening illness. Often the distinction is the client's individual perception of the illness. Clients with life-altering illnesses may try to convince themselves that nothing is wrong or deny the diagnosis. For some, this period provides time to come to terms with what is happening and to cope with the range of emotions they feel.

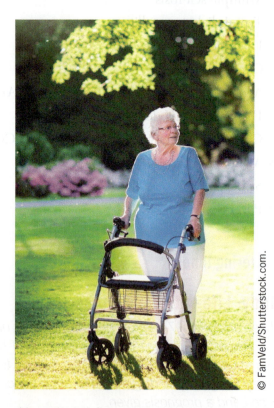

© FamVeld/Shutterstock.com.

FIGURE 10-1 A positive attitude influences the client's progression through a life-altering illness.

Professionalism

It cannot be said strongly enough that a health care professional will need to express warmth and caring, be genuine and honest with clients, listen and function with a sympathetic and empathetic ear, and assist clients in living their lives to the fullest. None of this can be accomplished unless a health care professional is comfortable with chronically ill individuals facing a life-altering or even a life-threatening outcome. There must be a non-judgmental attitude in all aspects of care. Review Chapter 4 for additional therapeutic responses.

Referring clients and their family members to illness-specific support systems such as the American Cancer Society and the Arthritis Foundation provides educational opportunities, emotional support, and access to others who know firsthand just what is being experienced. Medical social workers are also available to educate, instruct, and support clients and their families.

As the client processes the diagnosis, feelings of anger may be hurled toward the provider, health care professionals, or family members and friends. "How could you let this happen? I've been coming in for my annual physical exam. Why didn't you tell me about the risks?" Many clients fear the symptoms of the illness and the pain they may need to endure, but not death itself. Once the client reaches the acceptance stage of their prognosis, they worry about what will happen to their spouse, partner, and family, especially their children, once they are gone.

Stop and Consider 10.2

Review the life-altering illness case study and respond to the following questions.

1. What questions might come immediately to mind for Kyle and his parents?

2. Review Appendix A and identify therapeutic considerations for someone Kyle's age.

3. Can you think of any life-altering changes that may need consideration?

LOSSES FACED BY INDIVIDUALS WITH A LIFE-ALTERING ILLNESS

Persons who are chronically ill and who face a life-altering illness suffer many losses. They grieve their loss of good health, their independence, their body image, their lifestyle, and their sense of self-confidence. If they need constant medical care and attention, they may grieve their loss of privacy and modesty. Their daily routine is interrupted. Their financial security may be threatened.

Relationships change. Some relationships are lost; new ones are made. Established work and home roles are radically altered and daily routine is different. Plans for the future may be dashed. It may be impossible to participate in leisure activities once greatly enjoyed.

Sexual functioning may be altered. Health care professionals are equipped to discuss this alteration, but sadly it is not always done, because either the client or the health care professional feels uncomfortable in doing so. What is and is not possible with a disability should be discussed. What other forms of sexual expression might be encouraged if sexual intercourse is impossible is a question that needs to be addressed.

It is important to keep persons who suffer from a chronic or life-altering illness as comfortable as possible. Attend to their physical needs, teach them how to safely monitor their medications, provide them as much control as possible, answer their questions honestly, and also remember the concerns of family members. Embrace their culture as much as possible.

Stop and Consider 10.3

Review the opening case study and respond to the following questions.

1. What therapeutic actions do you see demonstrated by the surgeon in the opening case study?

2. Where would you put Billie on Maslow's Hierarchy of Needs during the various phases of her life-altering illness? (See Appendix A.)

3. What steps did Billie take to live a life that contributed to her well-being and to her family and society in general?

PSYCHOLOGICAL EFFECT OF LIFE-ALTERING ILLNESS

The basic personality of clients with life-altering illnesses may be changed significantly, depending on their psychological experiences. For example, the client who has always been thoughtful and kind may suddenly speak harshly or swear at those providing care. Or someone who is normally calm and loving may have periods of violence and hostility. Some clients who seem happy and upbeat most of the time may slump into a deep depression.

Personal relationships may also change during a life-altering illness. Your best friends may not be able to cope with watching you suffer, and may find excuses not to visit in order to manage their own guilt feelings. Some cope with their discomfort with life-altering illness by rushing around doing whatever, just to keep busy. Clients might prefer to simply have company, someone to just sit with them, to hold their hand, to listen. For some, it is difficult to touch or caress an ill person. The ill person may be the one to reject any close contact or relationships as well.

Setting personal goals for the client faced with a life-altering illness is an activity that distracts their focus away from the primary illness and toward therapeutic activities. Examples of personal goals may include the following:

- Establish goals to achieve something each week. This might include calling a friend to chat, taking a short walk, writing an email to a friend, or seeking an outlet through social media.

- Plan some things to look forward to in the long as well as the short term. Seeing a daughter married may be a short-term goal; seeing a grandchild born may be a long-term goal.

- Sign a physician's directive or living will, and a Durable Power of Attorney for Health Care.

- Update the last will and testament and arrange financial and personal affairs.

- Discuss any worries about pain and symptom control with medical professionals at an early stage.

- Learn about the illness and what to expect.

Health care professionals will want to be available to help clients deal with issues that are most frustrating and stressful. Help them problem-solve their day-to-day concerns and identify helpful resources.

MEDICATION CONSIDERATIONS

Medications are generally prescribed when treating life-altering illnesses. These medications may include, for example, analgesics for pain, sedatives for sleep, medications to treat the specific disease, antidepressants, tranquilizers, and the administration of oxygen. Health care personnel have been educated as to how and when to administer medications and understand the risks and side effects involved.

When the responsibility of administering medications is delegated to a family member, the situation can be problematic. The client or family member may feel the dosage is too strong and not give the prescribed amount. Or they may feel their loved one will become addicted to the medication if a large dose is given or if it is given too often. Many do not understand that it is important to take pain medication as it is prescribed, whether or not the client is in pain when the medication is due. Waiting too long to take the medication only renders it ineffective and causes unnecessary discomfort for the client. It is important for health care professionals to communicate to caregivers the need to strictly adhere to medical directions regarding medication. It is a good idea to maintain a medication journal providing the name of the medication, the dosage administered, the time given, and the initials of the one giving the medication. Other pertinent notes such as any side effects, pain level when administered, and taken with food may also be included in the notation.

CULTURAL INFLUENCES ON LIFE-ALTERING ILLNESS

Cultural

⊕ Modern technology has made it possible to live longer. We also live in a very mobile world with many cultures blended into our society. Cultural influences and preferences must be considered in health care. For example, should clients be told they have a life-altering illness? For most Americans, the answer would be yes; it is one of the basic patient rights to know. Other cultures, however, may value the family over the individual. Studies reveal that over half of the Mexican American population feel that clients should not be told the prognosis of their illness. This is also true of many Korean Americans. In Asian countries, such as China and Japan, it is customary for the provider to reveal the diagnosis only to the client's family. It is up to the family whether or not to share this with the client.

Some cultures consider it insensitive to tell clients they are dying. They feel it creates a sense of hopelessness and actually may hasten the dying process. Other cultures feel that the stress of knowing the condition would only cause the illness to worsen. Still others believe that only God knows when someone will die. The Hmong believe that to tell someone they are dying is to curse them. They wonder how you could know they would die unless you plan to kill them yourself.

It is important to remember that not all members of the same culture will make the same choices. For example, two Filipino families experienced the death of a family member. One of the families followed the traditional pattern of withholding the life-threatening diagnosis from the client. After the death, the family was pleased with their decision, as their loved one was able to live out her days without the added burden of knowing she was dying. The other family decided to tell the client the diagnosis. After the death, they felt satisfied with their decision, knowing that their loved one was able to make her final arrangements and say good-bye to family members. As health care professionals, we must be careful not to impose our own values on others, and not to stereotype cultures. Be aware of the patient's values, spirituality, and relationship dynamics. A teaching tool to help begin the process of spiritual assessment during the client interview uses the HOPE questions provided below (Anandarajah & Hight, 2001).

Professionalism

> **H:** Source of hope, meaning, comfort, strength, peace, love, and connection
>
> Where do you find comfort or hope in time of illness?
>
> When things are tough, what keeps you going?
>
> **O:** Openness
>
> Are you open to a spiritual component; a touch of the divine; recognition of a Supreme Being in your life?
>
> **P:** Personal spirituality practices
>
> Are there spiritual practices or beliefs that are important to you personally?
>
> **E:** Effects on medical care
>
> Are there ways that your personal beliefs affect your health care choices or might provide guidance as we discuss decisions about your health care?

Primary care providers will also tell you that they see a difference in their clients during surgery when they believe in prayer and are also surrounded by others who are praying for them. Clients may feel better prepared and ready for surgery and anticipate a divine presence during the surgical procedure and recovery process.

Stop and Consider 10.4

1. Would you want to be told you have a life-altering illness? Take time to do a self-assessment regarding your personal preference on whether you would want to be told.

2. Discuss cultures that would respond differently than you to the question, Should the client be told he or she has a life-altering illness?

3. Role-play using HOPE questions to assess spiritual beliefs and values.

The Therapeutic Response

- Understand the importance of cultural values and beliefs and do not stereotype.
- Be prepared for mood swings and realize that these may be part of the process of coming to terms with what is happening.
- Encourage open and honest discussion about emotions and feelings. Sometimes just listening and understanding demonstrates a therapeutic response.
- Include the client and family in discussions about a treatment plan when appropriate.
- Allow the client to make decisions whenever possible.
- Discuss any worries the client may have about pain or symptom control and their management.
- Educate family members about the illness and what to expect.
- Help the client and family members manage their stress.
- Deal with the present, the here and now.

SUMMARY

All illness is, at best, an inconvenience and can impact any age group. When the illness becomes chronic or life-altering, serious decisions must be made. Health care professionals will be called upon to help educate the client about the illness, what to expect, treatment regimens, and prognosis. It will be important for health care professionals to consider cultural differences when providing information and to not allow their personal biases and prejudices to hinder the therapeutic response. Expressing warmth and caring, being genuine and honest, listening, and encouraging clients in living their lives to the fullest are appropriate therapeutic responses. Providing community resources and illness-specific support system information is also helpful for the client and family members.

EXERCISES

Exercise 1

Choose two of the life-altering illnesses mentioned in this chapter and determine what support systems are available in your community for persons with these illnesses. List the full name, address, phone number, and Web site. Include when and where the support group meets and any other pertinent information.

Exercise 2

Using the Internet and your favorite search engine, look for information about three cultural values and beliefs that are different from your own regarding life-altering illness. Compile this information to be shared and discussed with classmates.

Exercise 3

Briefly respond to the following questions. This exercise can be used in small group settings or can be completed independent of others.

1. Your client has just been diagnosed with diabetes mellitus.

   a. What is your therapeutic response?

   b. What losses might the above client experience?

   c. What support systems might you suggest for your client to investigate?

2. Explore your feelings regarding the administration of pain medications and respond to the following.

   a. Would you want pain medications to be given to you if you were in severe pain that could last indefinitely?

b. Would you feel the same way if it were a loved one who was in pain?

c. Would addiction be a concern to you?

REVIEW QUESTIONS

Multiple Choice

1. Which is the best descriptor for acute illness?

   a. Lingers over a period of time

   b. Includes an experience of some stages of grief by the client

   c. Includes diseases such as COPD, cancer, and AIDS

   d. Has a rapid onset with severe symptoms and a short duration

2. Which is involved with curative care?

   a. Curing the illness and prolonging life

   b. Providing relief without curing

   c. Treating symptoms without curing

   d. Relieving or alleviating symptoms and providing supportive services

3. Which is the best descriptor of hospice care?

   a. Curing the illness and prolonging life

   b. Providing relief without curing

   c. Relieving anxiety and stress management

   d. Providing a program of palliative care and supportive services

4. Which of the following is true of psychological effects of illness?

   a. Personal relationships will not change.

   b. Learning more about the diagnosis only exacerbates feelings of concern.

   c. The client who is normally thoughtful and kind may speak harshly to caregivers.

   d. Life-altering illness always causes the client to slump into deep depression.

5. Which is the best descriptor for chronic illness?

   a. Symptoms linger over a period of time

   b. Has a rapid onset

   c. Has a short duration

   d. The diagnosis creates feelings of powerlessness and lack of control

FOR FURTHER CONSIDERATION

1. How do different types of illness (acute, chronic, and life-altering) impact the client and family members?

2. If you were diagnosed today with a life-altering illness, how would you feel and respond?

3. Do you feel there should be a different approach to medications for the client experiencing a chronic illness and the client whose death is imminent?

CASE STUDIES

Case Study 1

Suzanne, a hospice nurse, was assigned to manage the home care of Maria, a Spanish-speaking Mexican woman with metastatic breast cancer. Maria was receiving both chemotherapy and radiation; however, the cancer was progressing rapidly. Family members were close and loving and translated for Maria and Suzanne. Maria was desperately fighting not to let her disease upset normal family routines.

After 2 weeks of managing the case, Suzanne sensed an underlying strain. She felt the family was not coping as well as outward appearances indicated. Maria was choosing to compromise her comfort in order to maintain her traditional role in the family as wife and mother. She was becoming increasingly exhausted and withdrawn.

Suzanne decided to call in a bilingual/bicultural colleague to help assess the problem. Maria was able to talk more openly to the colleague when family members did not have to translate everything for Suzanne. Translating through her family members meant that Maria could not be as open and honest because she had to pretend she was doing well and maintaining normalcy.

1. Using the Internet, research the Mexican culture's views on family values and beliefs, and how these might impact life-threatening illnesses.

2. How would you rate Suzanne's evaluation of this situation?

Case Study 2

An older Iranian woman with a life-altering illness was slowly dying. The hospital staff felt that nothing could be done to improve her condition. Her son refused to sign the Do Not Resuscitate (DNR) order and insisted that everything possible be done to prolong his mother's life. Staff members could not understand this reasoning, and felt that it was causing needless suffering for the client.

1. Using the Internet, research the Iranian culture's family values and beliefs, and how these might impact life-altering and life-threatening illnesses.

2. Why is it important to understand other cultures' values and beliefs associated with health care issues?

3. How are cultural situations handled when the views of health care professionals and clients are different?

REFERENCES AND RESOURCES

Anandarajah, G. & Hight, E. (2001). Spirituality and medical practice: Using the HOPE questions as a practical tool for spiritual assessment. *American Family Physician* 63(1), 81–89. Retrieved from www.aafp.org/afp/2001/0101/p81.html.

Lindh, W. Q., Pooler, M. S., Tamparo, C. D., & Dahl, B. M. (2014). *Comprehensive medical assisting: Administrative and clinical competencies* (5th ed.). Clifton Park, NY: Cengage Learning.

Luckmann, J. (2000). *Transcultural communication in health care*. Albany, NY: Thomson Delmar Learning.

McCormick, T. R. (2014). Spirituality in medicine. Ethics in Medicine, University of Washington School of Medicine. Retrieved from http://depts.washington.edu/bioethx/topics/spirit.html.

Milliken, M. E., & Honeycutt, A. (2012). *Understanding human behavior: A guide for health care providers* (8th ed.). Clifton Park, NY: Cengage Learning.

Purnell, L. D. (2014). *Guide to culturally competent health care* (3rd ed.). Philadelphia: F. A. Davis.

Tamparo, C. D. (2016). *Diseases of the human body* (6th ed.). Philadelphia: F. A. Davis.

Chapter 11

The Therapeutic Response to Clients Experiencing Loss, Grief, Dying, and Death

CHAPTER OBJECTIVES

After completing this chapter, the learner should be able to:

- Define key terms as presented in the glossary.

- Describe Dr. George L. Engel's three processes for working through grief.

- Discuss Dr. Elisabeth Kübler-Ross's five stages of grief and dying.

- Identify at least six cultural differences in grief and death experiences.

- Identify five kinds of losses.

- Describe how age factors can influence grief.

- Contrast how men and women express grief.

- Explain the difficulties family members have in the grieving process.

- Compare anticipatory grief to dysfunctional and unresolved grief.

- List at least seven therapeutic responses to grief and death.

- Discuss the impact a physicians' directive has on dying and death.

- Research recent legislation in the right-to-die issue.

- Defend hospice as an alternative to the death event.

INTRODUCTION

Grief and how individuals face loss, dying, and death are very personal. Loss comes to us in many different avenues. Everyone has experienced grief from the loss of someone or something that had great meaning. Many have experienced the death of a significant person in their lives. Others express grief when suffering from a life-threatening illness or know someone who is. Dying is a process. Death is an event. Grief is a response.

KINDS OF LOSSES

World events afford everyone an opportunity to discover the kind of grief that accompanies loss. Devastating weather events such as the Haiti earthquake, the typhoon that devastated Taiwan and China and destroyed homes and lives, and drought and fires that burn farmland, forests, and residences provide ample opportunity to understand the kind of grief that comes from loss. Also, daily reports from war-ravaged countries show the loss of lives and the suffering of survivors. Check any form of news media and grief and loss will be reported.

Health care professionals will note that there are many additional kinds of losses that cause grief. They include (1) the loss of personal possessions

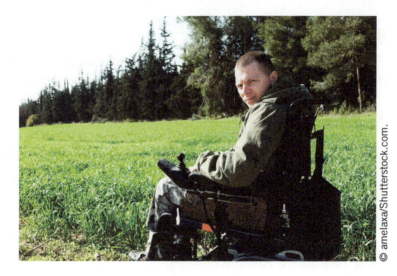

FIGURE 11-1 A wounded veteran enjoys the outdoors and ponders how his life has changed.

that have a great deal of meaning, such as a home destroyed by fire; (2) the loss of a familiar environment, such as a person who must move from a beloved area or who loses his or her job; (3) the loss of a significant other in a person's life—life partner, parent, child, close friend, family pet, etc.; (4) the loss of some part of the self—for example, the loss of a limb so commonly seen in today's wars (Figure 11-1), the loss of hearing or sight, or even the loss of psychological function such as memory, self-confidence, or respect and love; and finally, (5) the loss of life itself. In the loss of life, the concern is usually not so much from the death itself as it is from the fear of pain and the loss of control over one's life. For some, death is seen as a release or an entry into another life; for others, death and its separation and abandonment are seen as something to fear.

GRIEF

The experience of grief occurs when there is a loss of someone or something of personal value. Grief evokes an emotional response and may alter behaviors and cause unpleasant physical sensations. Emotionally the grieving person may feel sad, tired, depressed, angry, guilty, or anxious. Some have sleep disturbances, changes in appetite, experience forgetfulness, and cry easily. Many report feeling breathless, have little or no energy, and have tight feelings in the throat and chest. It is also known that the recently bereaved are vulnerable to illness. Two of the most well-known theories on death, dying, and the grieving process are presented here.

George L. Engel (1913–1999)

George L. Engel, MD, was a distinguished physician and teacher who devoted much of his career to investigating human relationships in the context of health, loss, and death. He identified three processes or stages of working through grief. They are (1) experiencing disbelief or shock over the loss, (2) realizing that the loss did occur, and (3) acknowledging the loss in a realistic manner.

During the shock and disbelief process, individuals may withdraw from social interaction or have difficulty carrying out normal daily activities. They may also have physical symptoms of sighing, shortness of breath, and being overly sensitive to noise. When individuals are finally beginning to realize the loss in the second process, feelings of guilt, anger, and frustration are common. Accepting the loss is the time when individuals have a desire to renew their lives and look to the future. They are able to face the loss in a realistic manner.

Elisabeth Kübler-Ross (1926–2004)

Another classic theory comes from Elisabeth Kübler-Ross, MD, in her book *On Death and Dying*. In the book, she presents five stages people may experience upon learning they are dying. In the years since 1969, and with much referral to these stages by health care professionals and others, the stages are now known as the "five stages of grief and loss."

1. *Denial:* This is the time when people deny reality.
2. *Anger:* This is the time when people express their anger and rage.
3. *Bargaining:* This is the time when people are willing to do anything to change what has or is happening to them. ("Let my son live, and I'll become a better person.")
4. *Depression:* This is a time of deep sorrow and feelings of aloneness when the loss is recognized.
5. *Acceptance:* This is the realistic acknowledgment of the loss.

Kübler-Ross also learned from her research that there was no order to the stages and that some people never make it through all the stages. In reality, these stages are now applied to all types of grief and loss. The research also recognized that individuals might pass through all the stages several times in doing their grief work.

CULTURAL INFLUENCES ON GRIEF AND DEATH

Cultural

A person's culture and heritage have a significant influence on the manner in which grief and death are met. Consider some of the following questions and examples for a better understanding of culture's role.

⊕ Do you place flowers on the grave for the dead person to smell, or do you place tools and food in the grave for the dead person's journey? Does your culture view death as a process the entire family embraces, or is grief an emotion to be borne alone? Would you and your family be most comfortable if you died in the hospital or in familiar surroundings at home? Is the hospital viewed as a place of death or a place for care and treatment?

In some cultures, end-of-life decisions are seldom made by the client, making hospital requirements that every person be asked about end-of-life choices upon admission difficult to achieve. Family members or the eldest child (in some cultures, the eldest son) may step in and make the decision, with the client's permission. Many prefer to die at home because of the belief that dying elsewhere means their soul will wander around with no place to rest. It is not permissible to discuss serious illness or death in some cultures. Some prohibit autopsy unless required by law and view organ donation as body mutilation.

The death ritual may be many different events (Figure 11-2). For some, it is a celebration of life; for others, the funeral is a social event that involves a long service, the body on display, and burial with a favorite possession. For others, it is a time of deep sorrow and weeping. Some families will delay the death ritual so that friends and family can travel long distances to arrive for the event. Others must bury their dead within 24 to 48 hours. In the Islamic faith, the dead person will be washed three times by someone of the same

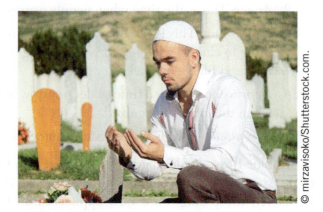

FIGURE 11-2 A follower of the Islamic faith praying for a dead relative.

sex and wrapped in white material prior to a prompt burial. In some cultures, it is appropriate to wear black as a sign of mourning; in others, white is worn. Some cultures will have family, friends, and loved ones keep watch around the clock over individuals who are dying or who have died; the idea is to never leave this person alone. Some release balloons at a grave; others sprinkle rice wine around it. Some family members in mourning cover mirrors in their homes to decrease focus on appearance; others wear black arm bands or white head bands. Some cultures bring gifts of money as well as food for the bereaved; others send sympathy cards.

Some cultures remember the dead on the anniversary of their death. Failure to do so would rob the living of rest. Some individuals return to gravesites yearly to clean the graves of weeds and debris, talk with the deceased, and share a picnic with family and friends. Others never return to the gravesite. Some are cremated, with ashes spread at sea or in a favorite place.

Health care professionals unaware of cultural differences may find themselves in uncomfortable situations, or feel embarrassed by saying or doing something that is inappropriate. It is important to obtain as much transcultural information as possible in order to respond and communicate in a therapeutic manner. Refer to the HOPE questions in Chapter 10.

FACTORS THAT INFLUENCE GRIEF

Case Study: Juliene's Christmas Grief

Juliene was going to visit her 85-year-old mother in an assisted-living apartment. It soon would be Christmas. She had with her a table-size decorated tree and a small nativity scene. She also had a small plate of the kind of fudge they made together during the holidays. Christmas was an important time for both of them; there were so many memories of decorating the Christmas tree and putting out the nativity. Juliene's mother was suffering from Alzheimer's disease and had been failing rapidly. When Juliene arrived, her mother seemed pleased to see her, immediately ate a piece of fudge, but ignored the Christmas tree and the nativity scene. Juliene put the tree on the table and placed the nativity underneath it, chatting all the while. Her mother seemed confused. Finally, she was able to say, pointing to the tree, "What is that?" As Juliene explained, it was clear that her mother did not understand. Juliene's eyes filled with tears as she realized she had lost another part of her mother. She cried all the way home.

A person's age will, in part, determine how one reacts to grief. *Infants* know only that there is a loss if someone is not there to feed, clothe, hold, and love them. *Toddlers* are confused and cannot distinguish animate from inanimate. Does the chair cry when it is broken? They feel anxious if someone is not there to care for them. *Children aged 3–5 years* believe that death is reversible. They think the dead person may just be sleeping; they are curious about life and death. *Children aged 6–10 years* are very curious about death. Is it cold in the ground? Can the dead move? What happens to the body? They want to do their own funeral ritual. This age group may dig up a dead pet to see what has happened to it. *Adolescents* have a fascination and a fear about death. They express the defense mechanisms of repression and denial and do not talk about a loss in peer groups unless it is the death of one of their own; then they dwell on it.

As common as divorce is in our society, children and adolescents are still devastated by divorce. They may feel very guilty about a divorce, blaming themselves and feeling like Mom and Dad do not love them anymore. Adolescents may need help from an older person they care about to cope with their grief. *Adults* sense that loss poses a threat to their pattern of living, perhaps their financial status, but are beginning to examine their own life and its meaning. *Older adults* grieve the aging process, grieve for their friends who have died, and fear a loss of independence.

Men usually have a more difficult time expressing grief openly, since they are mostly expected by society to be strong and supportive. *Women* generally have an easier time expressing grief, since they are perceived as needing the support of others. The opposite may be closer to the truth. It is fairly common in a retirement community for a man to follow his wife in death by only a few months, while a woman may pick up, change her life, and live many years after her husband has died. This may be in part because, traditionally, women throughout their lives are more likely to have a support network of friends to help them deal with their loss. A man more often than not sees his life partner as the person with whom he can talk and share grief. When that person is no longer present, it is difficult to grieve alone.

It has been said that the greatest grief comes from the loss of a child. Even if a person is 80 years of age and loses his or her 60-year-old child, the loss is as great as the loss of a young child. The loss of an unborn infant falls in this category also.

Everyone grieves at a different rate and in different stages. That is why it is so difficult for family members to help one another. One person may be in denial while the other is in depression; one is angry while the other is in acceptance. It is easy to "blame" the other person for no help or support.

It is usually impossible for spouses and partners to help each other in any way other than to share their love and their sadness. For this reason, it can be important to seek outside help in their grieving process.

Anticipatory Grief

Anticipatory grief occurs when individuals do part of the grieving process prior to the actual loss. People with life-threatening illnesses, people who are dying, and people who know they are going to lose a part of themselves begin the grief process early. This can be beneficial, if it helps individuals progress to a healthier state after the loss has occurred. It is not beneficial if individuals dwell upon the anticipated loss for extended periods. The most difficult grief work usually occurs when the relationship has been one with a fair amount of conflict, ambivalence, and unspoken messages. It is better to spend some time clearing up unfinished business and stating important messages to those close to you before a loss occurs. Many times grief is heightened by the fact that harsh words were spoken during the last encounter prior to death. Anticipatory grief simplifies the grieving process later.

Stop and Consider 11.2

Recall the case study where Juliene is visiting her ill mother before Christmas.

1. What kind of grief is Juliene experiencing? Explain.

2. Is her mother grieving? Why or why not?

3. What can be done to help Juliene through this process?

Dysfunctional and Unresolved Grief

Since everyone grieves at his/her own pace, and because there is really no one "right" way to grieve, caution must be used in labeling **dysfunctional** or **unresolved grief**. There are a few considerations to keep in mind, however, that may be helpful. Dysfunctional and unresolved grief can cause unexplained somatic responses, some stress-related medical diseases, and altered relationships with friends and relatives. An inability to cope with loss is disruptive to a person's physiological and psychological functioning. This process may be characterized by uncontrolled crying, hopelessness, helplessness, intense reactions lasting longer than 6 months, alterations in eating and sleep patterns, denial of loss, idealization of the lost person or object, and a constant reliving of past experiences.

Another kind of unresolved grief may be more difficult to resolve. This kind of grief comes when there is no finish or completion to the death event. A good example is the grief experienced by family members of individuals missing in action (MIAs). These people may know only that a body was not found and that their loved one is presumed dead. Crime victims whose bodies are never recovered, victims who are lost at sea—these, too, are examples of death that does not have a final event.

It is often beneficial for grieving family members to establish some kind of completion process. This might include a legal pronouncement of death, observing a death ritual, or planting a tree in the name of the person who is gone. Even pronouncing that the grief has ended and life is beginning again can be helpful.

LOSSES FACED BY INDIVIDUALS WITH A LIFE-THREATENING ILLNESS

Case Study: All Dignity Is Lost

Muriel was greeted by the infusion nurse who observed that Muriel appeared more pale, a little thinner than when she was last seen, and did not give the usual smile and "hello." They spoke quietly as the procedure began and Muriel revealed that she was having bouts of diarrhea and hoped she could make it through the hour and a half.

Stop and Consider 11.3

1. What might the nurse say to Muriel?

2. Will Muriel receive any special attention? If so, what and why?

The term *life-threatening* is used in this text as opposed to *terminal*. The reason should be obvious, but the use of *life-threatening* rather than *terminal* allows a place for hope and empowers a person to a higher degree of control over the circumstances. Individuals who receive the news that their illness is life-threatening realize that death may be imminent. This knowledge is different from the news that an illness is life-altering, since life-threatening implies that there may be only a little time left. When an individual who has been cancer-free for more than 5 years discovers the cancer has returned and is raging through several vital organs, there is a real threat to survival. There is no reprieve.

Cultural

 An individual's culture greatly influences his or her attitude toward a life-threatening illness. If clients are not in denial about a life-threatening illness, they may come to feel that there is an advantage in knowing that death is imminent. Individuals are more likely to make preparations for their final days. Are there people to say good-bye to? Do they need to seek forgiveness or forgive someone? Are financial matters in order? Are end-of-life decisions in place? Do they have any regrets? Is there anything they want to do, someplace they want to go, and someone they wish to speak to? If there is a project that needs to be finished, they may hasten to complete it. Some will tell friends and family of their diagnosis and that they do not have much time left. Others prefer that no one know the seriousness of their illness, so that no one will treat them differently. Some who know they are dying choose to do nothing differently because they try to live each day as if it might be their last. Others are glad to know that life is shortened because it allows them to put in place some action they had not taken the time to do previously. They find a new joy in life and may regret that they did not make the best of every day they had. Still others retreat into their private world to die, separating themselves from those they love, suffering alone—neither denying nor accepting the fact that life for them is drawing to a close. One thing is fairly certain, however: grieving will occur.

Case Study: All Dignity Is Lost   (*Continued*)

The unthinkable happened to Muriel. Without warning, loose and foul-smelling diarrhea began to run from her body. She called for help and two nurses came running. By the time she was released from the infusion pump, Muriel was quite a mess. She wept from embarrassment and loss of dignity.

Stop and Consider 11.4

1. How might the nurses help Muriel?

2. What can the nurses do to preserve Muriel's dignity?

THE RIGHT TO DIE

Legal

No matter in what context grief, dying, and death are discussed today, the topic of a person's right to die will likely surface. Advance directives and federal legislation in the Patient Self-Determination Act require health care institutions that receive Medicare and Medicaid reimbursement to establish written policies and procedures on advance directives, allowing individuals the right to identify clear choices in their death. At the risk of being too simplistic, there are at least two reasons why the courts and individual state constitutions have passed legislation on this issue.

The first reason is that physicians and health care providers are taught to preserve life. Death may be seen as failure. Allowing individuals to die, even when there is no hope for survival, is very difficult, even impossible for some. The second reason is that technology looks at death as another fatal disease to conquer at all costs. Medical technology has advanced much faster than has ethics. Without warning, dying individuals often get caught in a system in which technology has ultimate control.

One thing is certainly a result of all the publicity and discussion over an individual's right to die with dignity, to ask that no heroic measures be used, and to even seek assistance with death: individuals may be better informed and may have made decisions about their death prior to facing the event. These decisions may be reduced to writing in a legal document called a living will or a physician's directive.

Personnel in medical clinics may receive such directives from their clients. The directives should be discussed with their providers and filed with their medical records. When a person is hospitalized, a copy of the directive should be sent to the hospital. While the client's wishes should be respected and followed, health care professionals cannot be expected to act unethically or illegally. Any problems should be openly discussed to resolution.

A word of caution is given here. With increased numbers of private homes offering in-home care for older adults, a number of which are managed by individuals of various cultural backgrounds, individuals' living wills or physicians' directives are not always honored. Even when the caregivers have assured family members that such wishes will be followed, they often are not, due to the health care professional's own personal beliefs.

Dying individuals and family members may request that attending physicians keep the dying comfortable and free from pain. Some people who know they are dying may ask physicians if they can be given an injection or receive medication to end their life. The latter is more likely to occur when the dying process is slow, painful, debilitating, and likely to render a person unconscious. While refusing to commit an illegal act, physicians can be therapeutic at such a time by acknowledging and accepting the desperation felt, discussing with their clients how their pain can be managed, and assuring family members that suffering can be kept to a minimum.

Legal

Helping others to die is both a controversy and a debate in this country. Often the debate is fueled by those who have watched loved ones suffer immeasurably in their dying. Oregon was the first state to pass an assisted death law. Voters approved the law twice, but it faced a great deal of conflict both in and out of the court system. Finally, the U.S. Supreme Court ruled against John Ashcroft, the U.S. attorney at the time, to protect, by ballot, Oregon's right to choose assisted death. Aid in dying legislation is also now legal in Washington, Vermont, New Mexico, Montana, and California. As of 2015, at least 25 other states are currently considering legislation. The controversy continues, however, and with it comes the possibility of opposing legislation referred to as "health decision restrictions" that would make it difficult to withdraw nutrition and/or hydration from a permanently unconscious person. Legislation of this type is filled with emotion and faces both legal and ethical challenges on both sides of the issue.

Assisted death is the term used when someone provides the means for a person to end his or her life. *Euthanasia* is the term used when someone intentionally acts to terminate the life of a suffering individual. The Netherlands is the only country that allows both. Interestingly enough, individuals discussing their death choices while well and healthy will often propose such measures; however, the closer one is to death, the greater is the desire to delegate such decision making to professionals. As medical technology and science advance, the problem of how and when to prolong life will become more complex.

It may be helpful to remember that technology is a tool that does not have to be used. Life is not an idol to be worshipped. There is a time to die. Caring may very well be more important than curing.

In his book *Anatomy of an Illness*, Norman Cousins made this statement:

> Death is not the ultimate tragedy of life. The ultimate tragedy is depersonalization—dying in an alien and sterile area, separated from spiritual nourishment that comes from being able to reach out to a loving hand, separated from desire to experience the things that make life worth living, separated from hope.

HOSPICE

Many choose hospice services as a way to assure death without aggressive therapy or medications that may only prolong the inevitable. Hospice provides a multidisciplinary team of physicians, nurses, hospice aides, social

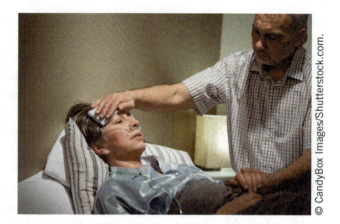

© CandyBox Images/Shutterstock.com.

FIGURE 11-3 A caring spouse giving comfort to his dying wife.

workers, bereavement counselors, and volunteers to tend to the needs of their clients and family members. The care is often provided at home, in a hospice center, or even in a hospital or nursing facility. Generally, hospice care is available when a diagnosis of terminal illness has been made and the prognosis is 6 months or less. The primary focus is comfort care and management of pain and symptoms when curative treatment is no longer desired (Figure 11-3). The emotional and spiritual needs of the client and family members are attended to and clients are encouraged to live each day as fully as possible. The goal of such services is dying at peace, in as much comfort as possible, and with dignity.

The Therapeutic Response

Responding therapeutically to individuals who are grieving a loss or facing death is a challenge. Recall the suggestions made in Chapter 10 related to the loss and grief that accompanies a life-altering illness. Generally, health care professionals are advised to keep their emotions distant from those they serve. The distance protects them from experiencing the same loss as their clients face. Such a distance cannot always be maintained, however, and perhaps it should not be. Medical providers who are too professional, appear aloof, or do not experience their clients' loss and grief serve only a part of their clients' needs. Recognizing the stages that clients might be experiencing and responding appropriately will go a long way to facilitate therapeutic communication. For instance, clients in the anger stage of loss may vent their anger toward you. Remember that their true anger is for the loss; it is not personal, toward you. Keep in mind the following:

- Accept individuals where they are and in what they are experiencing.
- Acknowledge individual cultural beliefs and values expressed during grief, no matter how different from yours.
- Listen to what is being said; listen to what is not being said.
- You cannot move a person out of denial. You can only help the person remain as close to reality as possible.
- Do not take any expressed anger personally. Be aware that you may try to avoid individuals who are angry, but avoidance is a roadblock to communication.
- Do not be embarrassed by clients' emotions or your emotions.
- Do not give false assurances or avoid discussing any problems that may be uncomfortable but must be addressed.
- Refer clients to counselors, clergy, attorneys, social workers, and/or hospice as appropriate.
- Answer clients' questions honestly and simply; they may forget your responses and ask again.
- Put information in writing for clients to refer to at a later time.
- Words may not be necessary, but if they are, it is most appropriate to say, "I am sorry. What can I do to help?"
- Honor clients' wishes with respect, even if they do not agree with your beliefs.
- Enable the dying person to remain independent as long as possible.
- Provide clients as much dignity as possible.
- Recognize that life-threatening illnesses take a great deal of energy. Help the individual conserve energy as much as possible.
- Demonstrate compassion and understanding.
- As a health care professional, do not view death as a failure of your profession. It is a part of the continuum of life.
- Allow yourself a "breather"—a time to draw away from the intensity of grief.
- Take care of yourself so you can take care of your clients.
- Leave the grief you experience in your professional setting where it is; do not take it home with you.

SUMMARY

Recall the stages or processes that individuals who are grieving are likely to experience. Respect the many cultural variances surrounding grief and death. If you are uncertain about what rituals are appropriate, ask your clients. They will be relieved to tell you their wishes. Learn to recognize what might be dysfunctional or unresolved grief and seek ways to assist clients through the process. Understand the legal guidelines in the state in which you are employed related to issues surrounding death and the observance of living wills, physicians' directives, clients' wishes, and assisted death.

Because health care professionals care for the sick and those who are facing death, they are likely to experience grief from the loss of a client or experience the grief expressed by clients because of some serious loss in their lives. Being present with these clients, listening to their grief, remembering that they are fragile at this time, and providing support and assistance as appropriate are the most therapeutic responses you can give.

On a personal note, it has been said that until you suffer a great loss, you cannot fully understand the depths of the sorrow and suffering that is called grief. If you have experienced heartbreaking loss, you are a part of the brotherhood and sisterhood of those who have felt the searing heat from the fire of deep sorrow. When you understand such loss, you know that suffering rips you open, but you also know that into that space flows compassion, if you will let it in.

Self-Awareness

In this process, take care of yourself and remember that you cannot be of help to others unless you are in touch with your own emotions. Seek advice and comfort from those around you, and allow time to process and recover from the loss. If you are employed in an environment where death occurs fairly frequently (long-term care facilities, oncology, or hospice), recognize that release from the stress caused by the loss is essential.

Finally, there is no need to ask yourself if you are strong enough to cope; you will be if you believe you can be. Strength comes from within. Remember the butterfly that comes wet-winged from its own chrysalis: from darkness into light; from confinement into freedom.

EXERCISES

Exercise 1

With a friend or classmate, discuss what kinds of choices you would make if you knew you were dying. What kind of medical care would you select? What would be most important to you? Write a brief report identifying your choices.

Exercise 2

Plan your funeral, memorial service, or death ritual. Discuss your choices with family members. Write a brief report describing your service.

Read the obituaries in the local newspaper. Then draft your own as you might see it in the newspaper.

Exercise 3

Either in discussion with others or by yourself, respond to the following:

1. A close friend was injured in a car crash that killed her 6-year-old daughter.
   You feel _____.
   You say _____.

2. A client shares with you as he leaves the clinic that he probably only has 6 months to live.
   You feel _____.
   You say _____.

3. Your partner tells you that he would choose assisted death over suffering in a terminal illness.
   You feel _____.
   You say _____.

4. You just attended a celebration of life for a dear friend's father who died at age 87.
   You feel _____.
   You say _____.

5. A 93-year-old has a mass in her left lung causing a fair amount of pain. The radiologist tells him it looks suspicious of cancer. The PCP says "At 93, let's just 'wait and watch.'"
   You feel _____.
   You say _____.

6. Your 6-year-old son digs up the family cat that he helped bury several weeks ago.
   You feel _____.
   You say _____.

7. As a hospice nurse, you observe your client is still receiving eight medications when only two were authorized by the physician and the family. You believe this is a cultural issue with the owners of the in-home care.

You feel _____.

You say _____.

REVIEW QUESTIONS

Multiple Choice

1. George L. Engel, MD, and Elisabeth Kübler-Ross, MD, both identify two common stages of grief. What are they?
   a. Anger and acceptance
   b. Depression and guilt
   c. Denial and acceptance
   d. Bargaining and denial

2. What factor most likely dictates death rituals?
   a. Religion
   b. Friends and family
   c. The eldest son
   d. Culture

3. What experience is often identified as the greatest loss?
   a. The death of a child
   b. The death of a spouse or significant other
   c. The loss of an arm, leg, or eye
   d. The loss of health

4. What is often the greatest fear a person has in facing life-threatening illness or death?
   a. The loss of respect and love
   b. The loss of some part of self
   c. The fear of pain and the loss of control over one's life
   d. The fear of separation and abandonment

5. Grief that is partially experienced prior to the actual loss is known by what term?
   a. Anticipatory grief
   b. Dysfunctional grief
   c. Unresolved grief
   d. Anxiety grief

FOR FURTHER CONSIDERATION

1. In the opening case study at the beginning of this chapter, what problems might Bob's family experience because he never moved from the denial stage of his illness?

2. It has been said that an individual who is dying and remains in denial never loses hope. Discuss.

3. Do you have a living will or a physician's directive? Why or why not? If not, who would make life-and-death decisions for you if you were unable to?

CASE STUDIES

Case Study 1

Jill Dawson was the mother of a beautiful young woman, Amy, who went to work for a social agency in South America after her college graduation. She loved working with the children in the little village where she and three others had been assigned. After a year in South America, Jon Peters, one of the men assigned to the same village, made sexual advances at Amy, but Amy was not interested. She tried to be diplomatic in her refusal, but it did not work. She reported her discomfort to agency headquarters and asked for a transfer. Their response was to tell her to "work it out."

One month later, the natives heard screams coming from Amy's hut. As they arrived at her door, they saw Jon Peters running out. He dropped a butcher knife as he rode away on his bicycle. Amy was inside with 14 knife wounds in her body. She died before they could get her to medical help. Jill received the dreaded call from the agency, which also informed her that Amy's assailant, one of the other agency employees, had been arrested for the crime. The murder trial was held in South America. Jon Peters was represented by the agency's lawyers, and was found innocent by reason of insanity. He was released into the custody of U.S. officials who accompanied him to the United States, where he was to be held in a mental institution.

Jill grieved for months. She grieved every birthday Amy might have had, she grieved the grandchildren she would never have, and she grieved the loss of a daughter. But, even through that grief, there was consolation in knowing that her murderer would not harm anyone anymore.

Twenty years later, Jill was approached by a writer who wanted to tell the story of what had happened to Amy. She agreed to be interviewed. The writer was sensitive and shared information with Jill. While she relived some of the horror, it helped her put into perspective what had happened. She found peace in telling her side of the story. Before the book was published, the writer visited her again. He said, "I don't want you to read this in my book; I must tell you myself. I found Jon Peters. He is living in Ottawa and works as an accountant for the federal government. He is married and has one daughter. He refused my interview requests. My research indicates no criminal record."

1. What can you learn from this story about grief? Does grief ever end? Why or why not?

2. Identify what Jill might have felt after learning the whereabouts of Amy's murderer?

3. If you were Jill, what might help you bring closure to your grief?

Case Study 2

Conner Leonard worked for Purges Manufacturing for 32 years. Along with four other men, he helped to start the company that designed and built products sold around the world. Purges Manufacturing grew and did very well, so well, in fact, that other companies wanted to buy it out. The company was sold three times in 12 years. Each time, Conner held onto his job. He was no longer helping in the design process, and had a more difficult time feeling pride in all the parts now made in another country where labor was cheap. Another buyout was looming. Conner knew he might be outsourced.

1. What kind of grief is Conner feeling? Justify your response.

2. Can you describe what it might be like to say good-bye to a job you loved, to a company you helped to build?

REFERENCES AND RESOURCES

American Bar Association. www.abanet.org.

Cousins, N. (1979). *Anatomy of an illness: As perceived by the patient.* New York: Norton

EMedicineHealth. Grief and Bereavement. www.emedicinehealth.com/grief_and_bereavement/article_em.htm.

Kiesling, S. (2006, September/October). Wired for compassion. *Spirituality and Health.* http://spiritualityhealth.com/articles/wired-compassion

Lewis, M. A., Tamparo, C. D., & Tatro, B. M. (2012). *Medical law, ethics, and bioethics for the health professions* (7th ed.). Philadelphia: F. A. Davis.

Purnell, L. D. (2014). *Guide to culturally competent health care* (3rd ed.). Philadelphia: F. A. Davis.

Zamichow, N. (2015, Spring). Be honest about the end of life. *Compassion and Choices.* Retrieved from https://www.compassionandchoices.org/userfiles/2015_Spring_MAG_Scott_web.pdf.

Appendix A
Theories of Human Growth and Development

INTRODUCTION

The following theoretical views introduce the medical health care professional to human growth and development. The theorists agree that personality and **cognitive** skills build upon each other as physical growth and maturity progress throughout the life cycle. The theories focus on different aspects of development; however, each of the theorists proposes progression through the stages in a sequential manner. This is not an exhaustive listing of developmental theorists, but will provide basic concepts and theories that represent major theorists in this area of study.

To appropriately care for clients, health care professionals must have knowledge of normal behavior for specific age groups and be able to interact on the client's level of understanding. The health care professional may also be involved in teaching primary caregivers how to help their clients through a particular crisis or stage of life.

OVERVIEW OF IVAN PAVLOV'S AND B. F. SKINNER'S BEHAVIORAL LEARNING THEORIES

Learning theorists recognize that laws of behavior can be applied at any age. Learning theory explores the relationship between stimulus and response. If a hand is waved in your face, the response is automatic—you blink. If you panic each time you pass the corner where you were in a serious accident, the response is learned.

Life is a continuing process of learning. One part of this learning is known as **conditioning**. Conditioning means that a particular stimulus or experience triggers a particular response.

Two theorists, Ivan Pavlov and B. F. Skinner, described how conditioning is critical to development. The two types of conditioning described are classical and operant. A brief discussion of these conditioned responses is helpful in further understanding therapeutic communication.

Ivan Pavlov, Behaviorist

Ivan Pavlov (1849–1936), a Russian scientist, is well known for his identification of the earliest and simplest form of learning. He identified **classical conditioning** in his famous dog experiment, which illustrates his theory. Pavlov knew that a dog salivated automatically as a reflex when there is food in its mouth. He presented food to the dog along with the ringing of a loud bell. Eventually the bell alone caused the dog to salivate—the learned response. To further illustrate, study the following example of classical conditioning.

Example of Classical Conditioning

Unconditioned stimulus —food	=	Unconditioned response —salivation
Conditioning —food and bell	=	Unconditioned response —salivation
Conditioned stimulus —bell	=	Conditioned response —salivation

Health care professionals often experience this classical conditioning, as seen in the small child who immediately begins to cry in fear when the assistant enters with a needle. The pain of the needle has been associated with the assistant so often that the child begins to cry just at the sight of the assistant. You may be able to relate similar responses. Some children become quite anxious at the smell they associate with the dental office. Others are afraid when they see someone in a white uniform.

Health care professionals remembering this conditioned response will consider various methods to help alleviate this fear and anxiety. Employees in a pediatric clinic might wear colors instead of white, or even consider uniforms with children's figures on them. Making the experience as positive as possible will help. The provider might carry a toy or an object of distraction. He or she is advised to spend some time with a child in a nonthreatening manner. The physical setting should include objects that delight a child. Many find a built-in aquarium beneficial. Others use appropriate children's media.

Even adults have conditioned responses that should be considered. A well-known cancer specialist, David Bressler, MD, purchases juggling bags for his cancer clients. His primary goal is to make certain his clients have something other than the cancer, the pain, and the difficult treatment to associate with him. This provider teaches the client something new about juggling on each visit. They often juggle their bags together. Of course, the added benefits are the laughter and the concentration on the juggling, which take the client's mind off the disease.

B. F. Skinner, Behaviorist

B. F. Skinner (1904–1990) formulated the learning model known as **operant conditioning**. Skinner and Pavlov agreed that classical conditioning explains some types of behavior. Skinner, however, believed that operant conditioning plays a much more important role.

The difference between classical conditioning and operant conditioning is that in operant conditioning, the response *precedes* the reward. For example, a rat pushes a lever and is rewarded with food. The food is pleasurable and useful, so the rat pushes the lever again. If the reward or consequence of pushing the lever is unpleasant, the rat will not repeat the behavior. Because a person's behavior is what brings the reward, this kind of conditioning may also be called **instrumental conditioning**.

Skinner believed that successful childrearing was accomplished through consistent rewarding of desirable behavior. If the behavior is followed by a pleasant reward or stimulus, the reinforcement is *positive*. If the behavior is followed by the removal of an unpleasant stimulus, the reinforcement is *negative*. Skinner believed that reinforcement was most effective if it was intermittent. Behavior would be rewarded most of the time, but not every time. Remembering this theory is helpful in therapeutic communication.

There are both *positive* and *negative reinforcements*. A positive reinforcement is something good or pleasant. A negative reinforcement is taking away the bad or unpleasant stimulus. The little girl who is upset and crying because of an injection receives a badge of courage from the assistant for the injection site. As the child is being told how brave she was, and the badge is put on, she begins to feel better and a smile creeps across her face. This is an example of negative reinforcement.

The father who rewards his son with an ice cream sundae because he did such a good job raking the lawn or the piano teacher who puts a gold star on a piece of music that was memorized are examples of positive reinforcement.

The reinforcement can be primary or secondary. A primary reinforcement is one that is basic and immediately satisfying, such as food. The reinforcement is secondary if the reward itself allows us to get something we want. An example of this is the allowance used as a reward that allows the child to go to the movies with a friend.

It is also helpful to distinguish between negative reinforcement and punishment. In punishment, an unpleasant stimulus is applied to discourage behavior. Punishment may be necessary, but the child can also learn to avoid punishment without changing behavior. For example, a student who receives a failing grade on an exam may avoid the circumstances and skip class rather than fail again. Such behavior requires attention from anyone who has control over the circumstances. The teacher must award the grade earned by the student, but should try to create a positive and encouraging atmosphere for the student, so they will study harder for the next test.

OVERVIEW OF SIGMUND FREUD'S PSYCHOSEXUAL STAGES OF DEVELOPMENT

Sigmund Freud (1856–1939), a Viennese physician, theorized that all human behavior is energized by *psychodynamic* forces, which he divided into three components. He called these forces the **id**, the **ego**, and the **superego**. In the mentally healthy person, these three forces work together cooperatively and enable the individual to realize fulfillment of basic needs and desires. When the three forces are at odds with one another, individuals are said to be maladjusted. His theory focused on *psychosexual development*, and emphasized that each stage must be conquered before progressing to the next stage.

The Id

Freud identified the id as a person's basic animal nature. It is primarily unconscious and is amoral. It is not governed by laws of reason or logic, and possesses no values or ethics. The id's primary function is to decrease pain and increase pleasure—also known as the **pleasure principle**.

In its earliest form, the id is a reflex response. For example, when a bright light falls on the retina of the eye, the eyelid closes and light is prevented from reaching the retina. The excitations produced in the nervous system by the light can then quiet down to maintain **homeostasis**.

An example of an internal reflex occurs during urination, when a valve in the bladder opens as the pressure on it reaches a certain intensity. The excitation or tension produced by the pressure ends as the contents of the bladder are emptied.

The id retains its infantile character throughout life. It cannot tolerate tension. It wants immediate gratification. It is demanding, impulsive, irrational, selfish, and pleasure-loving. It is the spoiled child personality. The pursuit of pleasure and the avoidance of pain are the only functions that count. It does not think; it only wishes or acts.

The Ego

The ego is the psychological force that is in touch with reality and mediates between the id and the superego. It deals with the outside world in a conscious fashion. The ego is governed by the **reality principle**, *reality* meaning that which exists. The goal of the reality principle is to postpone the discharge of energy until the actual object that will satisfy the need has been discovered or produced. For instance, we must learn to delay gratification (e.g., eating when we are hungry, sleeping when we are tired, and so on) until the timing or the situation is appropriate for fulfillment of our needs. This delay of action means that the ego has to be able to tolerate tension until it can be discharged in an appropriate form of behavior.

The institution of the reality principle does not mean that the pleasure principle is forsaken. It is only temporarily suspended. Eventually, the reality principle leads to pleasure, although a person may have to endure some discomfort while looking for reality.

The ego's lines of development are laid down by heredity and guided by natural growth processes. This means that every person has inborn potential for thinking and reasoning that come through experience, training, and education.

The Superego

The superego is the moral branch of the personality and represents the ideal rather than the real. It strives for perfection rather than reality or pleasure.

The superego is the person's moral code. It develops out of the ego as a consequence of the child's assimilation of his or her parents' or primary caregivers' standards regarding what is good and virtuous and what is bad and sinful.

The superego is made up of two groups, the **ego-ideal** and the **conscience**. The *ego-ideal* corresponds to the child's conceptions of what his or her parents or primary caregivers consider to be morally good. These standards of virtue are conveyed to children by rewards given for conduct that is in line with those standards. If they are consistently rewarded for being neat and tidy, then neatness is apt to become one of their ideals.

Conscience, on the other hand, corresponds to the child's conception of what his or her parents or primary caregivers feel is morally bad, as established through experiences with punishment. If children have been frequently punished for getting dirty, then dirtiness is considered to be something bad.

Freud's Erogenous Zones

Some regions of the body are more likely to experience tensions that can be relieved by some action upon the region, such as sucking or stroking. These areas are referred to as **erogenous zones**. Manipulation of an erogenous zone is satisfying because it affords relief from irritation (such as scratching relieves an itching sensation) and because it induces a pleasurable, sensual feeling.

The principal erogenous zones are the mouth, the anus, and the genital organs. Each of the principal zones is associated with the satisfaction of a vital need: the mouth with eating, the anus with elimination, and the sex organs with reproduction. Freud maintained that the erogenous zones are of great importance for the development of personality, since they are the first sources of tension the infant has to contend with, and they yield the first important experiences of pleasure.

The crux of Freud's theory is that each individual must successfully resolve the needs and conflicts of each stage in order to pass into the succeeding stage. The problem, however, according to Freud, is that many people do not reach the fulfillment of the genital stage and may fall prey to a variety of emotional symptoms and personality problems.

Table A-1 illustrates each of Freud's psychosexual stages.

TABLE A-1   **Freud's Stages of Psychosexual Development**

Psychosexual Stage and Age Range	Erogenous Zone	Sexual Activity
Oral (birth to 1 year)	Mouth, lips, tongue	Sucking, swallowing, chewing, biting, vocalizing
Anal (1–3 years)	Anus, buttocks	Expulsion and retention of waste products, toilet training
Phallic (Oedipus) (3–6 years)	Genitals	Recognize differences between sexes and become curious
Latent (7–11 years)	Genitals	Physical and psychic energy are channeled into the acquisition of knowledge and vigorous play
Genital (12 years and older)	Genitals	Puberty and maturation of reproductive system and production of sex hormones

OVERVIEW OF JEAN PIAGET'S STAGES OF COGNITIVE DEVELOPMENT

Jean Piaget (1896–1980), the renowned Swiss biologist and psychologist, wrote volumes on his research of child development. Piaget's *theory of cognitive development* states that motor activity involving concrete objects results in the development of mental functioning. For example, as an infant discovers his hand holding a rattle, he begins to recognize a sound that occurs every time he moves the hand holding the rattle. Therefore, reflex activity drops out as repetition produces a result that the infant observes: his activity begins to take on purpose. Eventually, the infant identifies the shaking rattle as a producer of sound. Later, he will realize that he is able to create the sound.

Cognitive refers to the ability to think and reason logically and to understand abstract ideas. Piaget states that, as cognitive development progresses, children gain insights, learn to solve problems, and are able to understand abstract concepts. Children's logic and modes of thinking are, initially, entirely different from those of adults. Piaget believed that cognition progresses through a process of adaptation: assimilation and accommodation. *Assimilation* involves the interpretation of events in terms of existing cognitive knowledge, whereas *accommodation* refers to changing the cognitive knowledge to make sense of the environment. Cognitive development consists of a constant effort to adapt to the environment in terms of assimilation and accommodation. Piaget felt that cognitive development came from the child's interaction with the environment.

Some believe that Piaget's theory is as important to cognitive development as Sigmund Freud's theory is to psychiatry. According to Piaget's theory of cognitive development, each individual needs to make sense of new experiences by relating them to existing understanding. Therefore, every child progresses through each stage of development in the same sequence; however, the timetable may vary from one child to the next. Cognitive development is a continuing process as more of life is experienced.

It should also be remembered that family, culture, personality, and socialization of the sexes may influence individual differences in cognitive development. Recognizing Piaget's developmental periods enables health care professionals to communicate on a level that matches a child's development and understanding. Sharing this information with parents who may be struggling to understand their child may also be beneficial.

Principles applicable to Piaget's theory of cognitive development include the following:

- Children will provide different explanations of reality at different stages of cognitive development.

- Providing activities or situations that engage learners and require adaptation (i.e., assimilation and accommodation) facilitates cognitive development.

- Learning materials and activities should involve the appropriate level of motor or mental operations for a child of a given age; avoid asking children to perform tasks that are beyond their current cognitive capabilities.

- Use teaching methods that actively involve the children's current challenges.

Piaget identified four stages or periods in which children progress in their learning. Table A-2 illustrates each of Piaget's cognitive development categories.

TABLE A-2   **Piaget's Stages of Cognitive Development**

Cognition Period and Age Range	Cognitive Activity	Therapeutic Approach and Desired Outcome
Sensorimotor Period (birth to 2 years)		Provide physical comfort and security to the child and educate the caregiver.
Stage 1 (birth to 1 month)	Sucking and innate reflex activity is paramount. The child does not differentiate between self and other objects.	Provide caregiver education and instruction regarding breast- and bottle-feeding.
Stage 2 (1–4 months)	The child begins to make distinctions, repeats simple actions, shows curiosity, and begins hand-to-mouth coordination.	Respond to the "social smile." Hold and support infant so that it feels secure. Infants can roll off the table, so never leave them unattended or take your eyes or hands off them.
Stage 3 (4–8 months)	The child experiences increased manipulation and control of objects; repeats rewarding activities and develops eye-to-hand coordination.	The infant recognizes familiar faces and voices, so include parent and/or primary caregiver in procedures where appropriate. Use caution in regard to what is within reach of infants.
Stage 4 (8–12 months)	In the period just prior to the first birthday, the child imitates and anticipates events more actively and shows a growing sense of organization of things.	Continue to formulate a positive experience with the infant. Use caution in regard to what is within reach or on the floor—everything goes into the mouth.
Stage 5 (12–18 months)	The child explores and experiments more and discovers new ways to get what he or she wants.	Smile when talking to infants of this age. Provide a warm and friendly atmosphere and be consistent. Safety measures must be exercised.
Stage 6 (18–24 months)	The child may have imaginary friends and is learning to speak words.	Infant is developing a memory and has some ability to think. Wearing colored uniform tops or jackets or buttons for interest may be helpful. Smile often and "talk" to the infant.

Cognition Period and Age Range	Cognitive Activity	Therapeutic Approach and Desired Outcome
Preoperational Period (2–6 years)	The child does not fully understand quantity, weight, length, and volume. Cannot follow or fully understand reality as it changes; thought is irreversible; cannot understand how something may change and then return to its original condition.	The child focuses attention on only one aspect of a situation. At this age child begins to think symbolically, as demonstrated through language formation, thinking of past and future events, and the ability to pretend and fantasize. Give simple commands and use games and imagery when appropriate.
Concrete Operations (7–11 years)	Child is able to classify objects by category; can focus attention on more than one situation at a time; able to distinguish length, quantity, and weight. Can consider another's point of view; understand that things can be reversed.	Communicate on a level that matches the child's development and understanding. Use praise and rewards to reinforce positive behavior. Allow the child to make decisions when making a wrong decision is not possible. (Should I see how tall you are first or how much you weigh?)
Formal Operations (12 years to adult)	This stage of adolescence is characterized by hypothetical, logical, and abstract thought processes. Most children can arrive at several possible solutions when given a problem. Long-term goals can be established. Understands symbols (i.e., political cartoons) and algebra. May be idealistic; challenge adult decisions and authority figures.	Help child make sense of new experiences by relating them with existing understanding. Communicate on a level that matches the child's development and understanding. Use praise to reinforce positive behavior.

OVERVIEW OF ABRAHAM MASLOW'S HUMANISTIC PSYCHOLOGY

Abraham Maslow (1908–1970) is considered the founder of humanistic psychology. Maslow was not opposed to other theorists; he simply regarded his work as an extension of modern trends in psychology. He is well known for his **Hierarchy of Needs**, which is often used to illustrate motivating forces.

While working with monkeys early in his career, Maslow noticed that some needs took precedence over others. For example, if the monkeys were

TABLE A-3   **Maslow's Hierarchy of Needs**

Progression of Need Level	Examples of Specific Needs
Physiologic needs	Oxygen, water, protein, electrolytes, minerals, and vitamins
Safety needs	Safe environment; stability; protection; freedom from fear and anxiety; need for structure, law and order, and limits
Love and belonging needs	Need to give and receive affection; desire to marry, have a family, be part of a community
Esteem needs	Basic need for a stable, healthy respect for self and others; Desire for achievement, strength, confidence, recognition, prestige, reputation, status, and fame
Self-actualization	Achievement of potential—doing what you are truly fitted for

hungry and thirsty, they would tend to seek water first. You can do without food for weeks, but you can only live without water a few days. If someone had a chokehold on you and you could not breathe, what would be most important? Breathing, of course. Maslow also concluded that sex is less powerful than food, thirst, and air to breathe. No one has ever died from not having sex.

Maslow believed that individuals move back and forth from one need to another, depending on the circumstances present at the time. He also demonstrated that development continues throughout the life cycle. Table A-3 illustrates Maslow's Hierarchy of Needs.

OVERVIEW OF LAWRENCE KOHLBERG'S STAGES OF MORAL DEVELOPMENT

Lawrence Kohlberg (1927–1987) was a psychologist who was born in Bronxville, New York, and served as a professor at Harvard University, where many of his studies on moral development were completed.

Kohlberg developed a theory that moral development is dependent on the thinking and problem solving stimulated in the child. The theory claims that individuals acquire a sense of justice through a sequence of stages related to cognitive development. The stages are closely parallel and are built on Piaget's theory and research.

Progress from one stage to another depends on a person's cognitive development and the opportunity to be exposed to different ideas and experiences. Standards change as society changes. As children grow older, however, discipline given in love seems to be more effective when encouraging moral development than is discipline that is aggressive and controlling.

Table A-4 illustrates the six identifiable levels of moral development according to Kohlberg.

TABLE A-4   **Kohlberg's Levels of Moral Development**

Moral Development Level and Orientations	Behavior	Moral Dilemma
Preconventional Level		
Obedience and punishment orientation	To do good is to avoid punishment.	Individuals in this level judge the morality of an action by its direct consequences.
Self-interest orientation	You be good to me and I'll be good to you.	
Conventional Level		
Conformity orientation	Child learns to be a "good" boy or girl because there is value in doing so.	Moral behavior is what is accepted and approved by others. Approval becomes more important than reward.
Law-and-order orientation	Child learns the importance of obeying the law and social standards.	Law and order as well as fixed rules are recognized, either by religion or social order or both.
Postconventional Level or Principled Level		
Social contract orientation	Actions are determined by individual rights or standards, such as the described laws and the U.S. Constitution.	Individuals in this reasoning level think actions are wrong if they violate their ethical principles. Laws may be changed when necessary as long as there is agreement.
Principled conscience orientation	Morality becomes individual principles that are logical, comprehensive, and consistent. Justice and equality of human rights, respect, and worthwhile life is recognized. Universal ethical principles are established.	

OVERVIEW OF ERIK ERIKSON'S EIGHT STAGES OF PSYCHOSOCIAL DEVELOPMENT

Erik Erikson (1902–1994) was born in Frankfurt, Germany. His adolescent years were spent wandering through Italy, his young adulthood in Austria working with Freud, and his later life in the United States.

Erikson's psychosocial theory is an approach to personality that extends the Freudian psychosexual theory. Like Freud, Erikson taught that psychological development is a continuous process; each phase or stage is part of a continuum throughout the life cycle. Each developmental stage presents a problem or crisis that the individual must face and master. These **psychosocial crises** are conflicts between a person and society or social institutions. They are the motivating forces behind the individual's behavior. Resolution of each life crisis enhances a person's ability to meet the next crisis and is characterized by hypothetical, logical, and abstract thought processes. Table A-5 illustrates Erikson's eight psychosocial crises.

TABLE A-5   **Erikson's Stages of Psychosocial Development**

Psychosocial Crisis and Age Range	Growth and Development	Therapeutic Approach and Desired Outcome
Trust versus Mistrust Infancy		Provide physical comfort and security to the child and educate the caregiver.
Birth to 4 weeks	*Motor Development:* Visual fixation (stares at windows and ceiling); eyes follow bright moving objects; head sags when unsupported; makes crawling movements when prone. *Physical Growth:* Gains 5–7 ounces weekly and grows one inch monthly (for 6 months). *Vocalization:* Cries when hungry or uncomfortable, making throaty sounds. Tries to communicate pain or discomfort.	Health care professional should smile and use a pleasant, calm voice when speaking with infant caregivers. Encourage caregivers to verbalize their feelings and concerns and respond to each inquiry. Educate caregiver in understanding that the infant is dependent upon others and how to interpret ways in which the infant makes known those needs. Hold and support the infant so that it feels secure.

Psychosocial Crisis and Age Range	Growth and Development	Therapeutic Approach and Desired Outcome
2 months	*Motor Development:* Eyes are better controlled; can turn body from side to back; can hold head erect, in midposition. *Physical Growth:* Growth patterns continue; posterior fontanel closed. *Vocalization:* Knows crying will get attention; crying becomes differentiated—for hunger, pain, attention. *Socialization:* Begins to respond to attention by expressing a "social smile" in response to others.	Respond to the "social smile." Hold and support the infant so that it feels secure. Remember infants of this age can roll off a table or counter, so never leave them unattended or take your eyes or hands off them. Mobiles over the examination table create a pleasing atmosphere for the infant.
3 months	*Motor Development:* When prone, infant will rest on forearms and keep head midline; discovers and stares at hands; plays with hands and fingers; able to place hand or object in mouth at will. *Vocalization:* Babbles and coos, laughs aloud; shows pleasure in making sounds; makes initial vowel sounds. *Socialization:* Recognizes parent or primary caregiver.	The infant recognizes familiar faces and voices, so include parent and/or primary caregiver in procedures where appropriate. Use caution in regard to what is within reach of infants, as they are much more active at this stage.
4 months	*Motor Development:* Holds head up; can turn body from back to side; recognizes familiar objects; sits with adequate support. *Physical:* Drools (does not know how to swallow saliva); deciduous teeth appear. *Vocalization:* Vocalizes socially (coos when talked to)—very talkative. *Socialization:* Enjoys having people close by; initiates social play by smiling.	Continue to formulate a positive experience with the infant. Use caution in regard to what is within reach or on the floor—everything goes into the mouth.

(*continues*)

TABLE A-5   **Erikson's Stages of Psychosocial Development (*continued*)**

Psychosocial Crisis and Age Range	Growth and Development	Therapeutic Approach and Desired Outcome
6 months	*Motor Development:* Reaches for objects; grasps objects with whole hand; can hold two objects—one in either hand; can pull self to sitting position; hitches for **locomotion**. *Physical:* Doubles birth weight; continues to gain 3–5 ounces weekly and grows one-half inch monthly. *Vocalization:* Vocalizes displeasure as well as several distinguishable syllables; cries easily. *Socialization:* Begins to recognize strangers.	Smile when talking to infants of this age. Provide a warm and friendly atmosphere. Safety measures must be exercised.
8 months	*Motor Development:* Bounces and bears some weight when held in standing position; discovers feet; hand–eye coordination is perfected; sits alone; displays exploratory behaviors with food. *Vocalization:* Makes polysyllabic vowel sounds; imitates speech sounds. *Socialization:* Shows fear of strangers and affection for family members.	The infant is developing a memory and has some ability to think. Wearing colored uniform tops or jackets or buttons for interest may be helpful. Smile often and "talk" to the infant.
10 months	*Motor Development:* Crawls and creeps; raises self to sitting position; sits alone; preference for use of one hand; manipulates objects; can hold bottle. *Vocalization:* Says one or two words; is able to initiate expression and gestures. *Socialization:* Pays attention to his or her name; plays simple games (pat-a-cake, peek-a-boo); responds to adult anger (tone of voice).	Involve child in simple games; be aware of the tone of voice used; when child is eating, use care to prevent choking.

Psychosocial Crisis and Age Range	Growth and Development	Therapeutic Approach and Desired Outcome
12 months	*Motor Development:* Stands alone for a moment; walks with help; can sit from standing position without help; can pick up food and transfer to mouth; cooperates in dressing. *Physical:* Triples birth weight; doubles birth length. *Vocalization:* Uses expressive jargon; recognizes meaning of "no-no." *Socialization:* Still egocentric; shows emotions (jealousy, affection, anxiety, and anger); responds to music.	Use praises and rewards to reinforce positive behavior. May play music in examination room. Allow the child to help dress after a procedure.
12–15 months	*Motor Development:* Walks alone; can release objects at will; tells parent or primary caregiver "I do it"; gets into things; has one-directional thinking—mine, no-no. *Physical:* **Babinski and Landau reflexes** disappear. *Vocalization:* Points to indicate wants. *Socialization:* Shares emotions; enjoys being center of attention.	The key element at this stage of development is safety. Use large blocks, stuffed toys that are washable, and cloth books in the reception area and examination room. Do not keep children and parents waiting long; excessive waiting encourages anxiety.
Autonomy versus Shame and Doubt Toddler	The child's energies are directed toward the development of physical skills, including walking, grasping, and rectal sphincter control.	Encourage and praise their physical accomplishments.
18–24 months	*Motor Development:* Walks up and down stairs; opens doors; turns knobs; uses spoon without spilling; helps undress self; can jump. *Vocalization:* Knows 200–300 words; begins to use short sentences. *Socialization:* Obeys simple commands; uses word "mine" constantly; enjoys parallel play (health care professional plays with a puppet while the child also plays with a puppet).	Use simple commands such as "roll over" and "give me the book"; reward acceptable behavior with hugs and stamps on the hand.

(continues)

TABLE A-5   **Erikson's Stages of Psychosocial Development (*continued*)**

Psychosocial Crisis and Age Range	Growth and Development	Therapeutic Approach and Desired Outcome
2–3 years	*Motor Development:* Feeds self well; can undress self; walks backward; begins to use scissors. *Physical:* Has full set of 20 deciduous teeth. *Vocalization:* Knows 900 words. *Socialization:* Negativism grows out of child's sense of developing independence; rituals are important.	Develop a consistent routine for office visits; provide rewards for positive behavior; talk to the child directly as much as possible.
Initiative versus Guilt Preschool age	The child continues to become more assertive and to take more initiative.	Foster initiative to master new tasks.
(3–6 years)	*Motor Development:* Dresses self (buttons shirt and ties shoelaces); climbs and jumps well. *Physical:* Growth is relatively slow (gains less than 5 pounds per year and grows 2–2½ inches per year). *Socialization:* Talks to imaginary friends; can be given simple explanations as to cause and effect; still needs security of parent's or primary caregiver's presence; initial need to be accepted by others outside the family; strong motivation to measure up.	Give simple explanations and short, simple commands. This age responds well to drawings and play. May give a pretend injection to doll and explain, "This will hurt for a minute. It will help you feel better so you can play."
Industry versus Inferiority Grade school years	The child must deal with demands to learn new skills or risk a sense of inferiority, failure, and incompetence.	Productivity and mastery of skills.
(6–11 years)	*Motor Development:* Coordination is refined; begins to develop independence; likes to bathe self without assistance. *Physical:* Height increases proportionally to weight gain; begins to lose baby teeth; acquires first molars.	Provide encouragement and praise where appropriate. Encourage self-esteem. Explain procedures at the child's level of understanding. Provide choices where appropriate: "Should I check how well you can see first or how well you can hear?"

Psychosocial Crisis and Age Range	Growth and Development	Therapeutic Approach and Desired Outcome
	Socialization: Begins to take responsibility for own actions; begins to accept authority outside the home; uses the telephone; works for acceptance; has to be good at something or feels inferior; no interest in the opposite sex.	
Identity versus Role Confusion Adolescence	The teenager must achieve a sense of identity in occupation, sex roles, politics, and religion.	Ability to be oneself.
(12–18 years)	*Motor Development:* Awkward. *Physical:* Females—menstruation begins; axillary and pubic hair becomes coarser and darker; increased development of breasts. Males—grow pubic and facial hair; growth spurts in height; shoulders broaden; voice changes; axillary hair develops; production of spermatozoa, nocturnal emission may occur. Both males and females—sebaceous glands on face, back, and chest become more active. *Socialization:* Increased interest in the opposite sex; concerned with morality, ethics; peer group important; emancipation from family begins.	Peer importance is critical. Provide privacy and remember this group is very modest. They have a fear and concern regarding future changes in body image. Will this procedure or process impact future activity levels?
Intimacy versus Isolation Early adulthood	The young adult must develop intimate relationships or suffer feelings of isolation.	Capacity for affiliation and love.
(19–40 years)	This group is interested in the development of a career, searching for a mate, and establishing a home and family. *Physical:* In general, experiencing good health and at their peak. Usually only routine examinations or emergency care for an injury or illness is all that will be needed.	At this stage individuals are self-confident and able to make rational decisions regarding their health care. Provide options and describe the benefits and expectations of good health care.

(continues)

TABLE A-5   Erikson's Stages of Psychosocial Development (*continued*)

Psychosocial Crisis and Age Range	Growth and Development	Therapeutic Approach and Desired Outcome
Generativity versus Stagnation Middle adulthood (40–65 years)	Each adult must find some way to satisfy and support the next generation. This can be the most productive period, as individuals are making and discovering new things. Usually established socioeconomically and do not have to struggle. Begin to think of charity; give back to their parents and community. *Physical:* Health maintenance is important during this stage. Routine examinations and procedures need to be evaluated regularly. A balanced diet and exercise program should be maintained. Attention should be given to stress levels and how to cope with stress in life experiences.	Concern for the succeeding generation. If these clients are not fulfilled, they will feel empty and dissatisfied. They either feel good about the past or they despair. Often they will brag of past accomplishments, reasserting worth. Listen to what they have to say. Provide health care choices when appropriate.
Ego-Integrity versus Despair Late adulthood (65 to death)	These individuals are beginning to think of retirement or have retired, looking back on their lives and accomplishments. They may be afraid to die or may feel they have not lived life to its fullest. *Physical:* The body or mind or both may begin to fail. Body functions begin to decrease and/or malfunction.	Reflection on and acceptance of one's life; feeling fulfilled. Give these individuals a firm handshake and eye contact; address them by their full name and title; ask their opinion; allow them to make decisions regarding their health care if possible. Do not refer to them using endearing terms such as "dear," "sweetie," or "honey."

EXERCISES

Exercise 1

A client comes to the dental office in obvious pain and discomfort from a severely abscessed tooth. The client remarks, "I couldn't sleep, I can't eat, and I couldn't go to work today."

Which of Maslow's stages most accurately describes the client? What action should the health care professional take to assist this client?

Exercise 2

As you reflect upon moral development and the information in Appendix A, you have probably been reminded of your own moral development. In a short report to be shared with your instructor, identify the individuals who were influential in your moral development. What is it that these people modeled for you? What other influences have been instrumental in your moral development? Try to identify *only five* beliefs you have about morality. You may have many more; however, try to determine which five would be the most important. Compare your list of five with others in class. Discuss what might cause these differences. Are the differences related to models? Culture? Religion?

REFERENCES AND RESOURCES

Frisch, N. C., & Frisch, L. E. (2010). *Psychiatric mental health nursing* (4th ed.). Clifton Park, NY: Thomson Delmar Learning.

Mandleco, B. L. (2004). *Growth and development handbook: Newborn through adolescent*. Clifton Park, NY: Thomson Delmar Learning.

Smith, L. (2000). A brief biography of Jean Piaget. In *Jean Piaget Society: Society for the study of knowledge and development*. Retrieved from www.piaget.org/aboutPiaget.html.

Thornton, S. P. (n.d.). Sigmund Freud. In *The Internet encyclopedia of philosophy*. Retrieved from www.iep.utm.edu/freud/.

Appendix B
Defense Mechanisms

INTRODUCTION

The term **defense mechanisms** has been defined as behavior that is used to protect the ego from guilt, anxiety, or loss of esteem. An individual wishing to block an emotionally painful experience may, subconsciously or consciously, use a defense mechanism. This enables the individual to put a problem on hold until sufficient time has elapsed to work through the situation and arrive at a solution, or come to terms of acceptance.

The use of defense mechanisms may be healthy or unhealthy. It may be considered an unhealthy approach if the problem is never resolved. Behavior resulting from the use of defense mechanisms may be inappropriate in later developmental stages. An example might be the child who throws a temper tantrum in an effort to get the parents' attention. Then, during early school years, this same child becomes the class clown in order to seek attention from those in authority.

The use of defense mechanisms is difficult to analyze, since it is the motive behind the behavior that characterizes the various mechanisms and gives them their individuality. Some mechanisms may be used to provide time to adjust to and accept a problem, while others may be used to cope with or survive a situation. Some commonly used defense mechanisms are described here.

Compensation is consciously or unconsciously overemphasizing a characteristic to compensate for a real or imagined deficiency. For example, the young boy whose physical stature may keep him from being a football star may compensate by achieving an academic award.

Denial is the unconscious refusal to acknowledge painful realities, feelings, or experiences. Denial offers a temporary escape from an unpleasant event. For example, when a laboratory report comes back positive and the client is told, they may express denial by saying, "There must be a mistake!"

Displacement is shifting the emotional element of a situation from a threatening object to a nonthreatening one. An example is the client who is very angry with the provider for not explaining a procedure completely. When the client leaves the office, the door is slammed really hard, when in reality, the provider is being "slammed."

Projection is attributing one's own thoughts or impulses to another individual as if they had originated in the other person. Usually negative or unacceptable feelings or urges are projected. From this perspective, every bad choice made is someone else's fault. For example, the drug-dependent client who blames someone else because there is no money to pay the rent or buy food.

Rationalization is the mind's way of justifying behavior by offering an explanation other than a truthful response. It is often used to save face or avoid embarrassment. There is usually some grain of truth in the explanation. For example, the client told by the physical therapist to exercise the neck several times a day for 5 minutes may respond with an excuse such as, "I couldn't do the exercise that often because I had to go to work." The client could have done the exercise seated at a desk.

Regression is an attempt to go back to an earlier stage of development to escape fear, anxiety, or conflict. Toddlers who have been toilet-trained for a year or two when a new baby arrives in the household may become anxious or feel displaced and regress to soiling themselves again.

Repression is the unconscious blocking from awareness material that is threatening or painful. It is the mind's way of forgetting or experiencing temporary amnesia until it can cope with an overwhelming circumstance. Clients with posttraumatic stress disorder may use repression to deal with things too painful to face.

Suppression is the conscious or unconscious attempt to keep threatening material out of consciousness. It is deliberately refusing to acknowledge something that causes mental pain or suffering. An example would be the failure to remember a significant childhood event, such as the death of a grandmother.

Sublimation is redirecting a socially unacceptable impulse into socially acceptable behavior. For example, the artist who expresses sexual impulses in sculpture or paintings is sublimating.

Undoing is canceling out a behavior or trying to make amends. The individual is trying to make up for an inappropriate behavior and the guilty feelings that accompany the act. An abusive person often showers the abused with gifts after the abusive event, hoping to "undo" the unacceptable behavior.

EXERCISES

Exercise 1

Review the list of defense mechanisms. Identify the one you use most often. List an instance when you used it in the last 2 weeks, and describe the results.

Exercise 2

Enjoy an evening watching your favorite television programs. List the defense mechanisms you observe and describe how these were used and the results of their use.

REFERENCES AND RESOURCES

Frisch, N. C., & Frisch, L. E. (2010). *Psychiatric mental health nursing* (4th ed.). Albany, NY: Thomson Delmar Learning.

Lindh, W. W., Pooler, M. S., Tamparo, C. D., & Dahl, B. M. (2014). *Comprehensive medical assisting: Administrative and clinical competencies* (5th ed.). Albany, NY: Thomson Delmar Learning.

Milliken, M. E. (2012). *Understanding human behavior: A guide for health care providers* (8th ed.). Albany, NY: Thomson Delmar Learning.

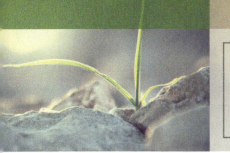

Glossary

Acupressure Needles are not used; only pressure is applied on the points using fingers, palms, elbows, or feet; believed to restore health and balance. See *Acupuncture*.

Acupuncture Piercing the skin with extremely thin, sterile needles at the point of one of the 365 points along the 12 meridians of the body.

Acute Having rapid onset, severe symptoms, and a short course.

African American Venacular English (AAVE) Colloquially know as Ebonics, or Black English.

Allopathic medicine A system of medical care using remedies to counteract disease and illness.

Anticipatory grief Grief experienced prior to the actual loss.

Anxiety A vague, uneasy feeling of discomfort or dread accompanied by an autonomic response.

Autonomic nervous system The part of the nervous system that controls involuntary bodily functions.

Autonomy versus Shame and Doubt Erikson's psychosocial crisis from 18 to 24 months of age.

Babinski reflex A reflex action of the toes, indicative of abnormalities in the motor control pathways.

Bias A slant toward a particular belief.

Biopsychosocial Pertaining to the biological, psychological, and social aspects of disease.

Blog A Web site that is run by an individual or a group, is regularly updated, and generally is informal or conversational in style.

Bullying Unwanted aggressive behavior that invokes a real or perceived power imbalance.

Child abuse Deliberate harm or injury of a child by a parent or caretaker.

Chronic Illness with a long duration.

Classical Conditioning A procedure in which a conditioned stimulus, through repeated pairings with an unconditioned stimulus, comes to elicit the conditioned response. (For example, a dog is given food when a bell is rung. The dog's response is to salivate. After repetition, the dog will salivate when the bell is rung, even when it is not given food.)

Clichés Patterned responses; trite expressions; empty, meaningless phrases.

Clustering Grouping of gestures, facial expressions, and postures into nonverbal statements.

Cognitive The ability to think and reason logically and to understand abstract ideas.

Cognitive behavioral therapy (CBT) Form of psychotherapy used to treat depression and other mental disorders.

Compensation Consciously or unconsciously overemphasizing a characteristic to compensate for a real or imagined deficiency.

Concrete Operations Piaget's cognition period from 7 to 11 years of age.

Conscience The part of self that judges the self in terms of values and activity; the superego.

Conventional level Kohlberg's theory that moral behavior is what is accepted and approved by others.

Culture A pattern of many concepts, beliefs, values, habits, skills, instruments, and art of a given group of people in a given period.

Cupping Glass, bamboo, or pottery cups are placed on the skin to create a suction; believed to increase blood flow and healing to area of discomfort.

Curative care Health care practices that treat clients with the intent of curing them.

Defense mechanisms Behavior that protects the psyche from guilt, anxiety, or shame.

Denial Unconscious refusal to acknowledge painful realities, feelings, or experiences.

Detoxification A period of time in which to rid the body of the abused substance.

***Diagnostic and Statistical Manual of Mental Disorders* (DSM)** Published by the American Psychiatric Association. Used by mental health care professionals for a wide range of purposes, including clinical, research, administrative, and educational.

Dialect The form of a spoken language peculiar to a region, social group, etc.

Displacement Shifting the emotional element of a situation from a threatening object to a nonthreatening one.

Distress Considered to be unhealthy stress.

Doshas Biological energies in the body and mind that provide a blueprint for health; Ayurveda theory.

Doula A woman trained in assisting another during and after childbirth.

Drug Enforcement Agency (DEA) Federal agency that identifies and enforces controlled substance regulations.

Dysfunctional grief Grief that is unresolved.

Ego The psychological force that is in touch with reality and mediates between the id and the superego.

Ego-ideal Corresponds to the child's conceptions of what the parents or primary caregivers consider to be morally good.

Ego-Integrity versus Despair Erikson's psychosocial crisis from age 65 to death.

Elder abuse Deliberate harm or neglect inflicted on someone who is age 60 or older.

Erogenous zones Body areas that provide pleasurable sensations.

Ethnocentrism The belief that one's own group or culture is superior to all other groups or cultures.

Eustress Good stress; optimal amount of stress that helps to promote health and growth.

Food and Drug Administration (FDA) Federal agency responsible for protecting public health and safety of drugs, biologicals, medical devices, nation's food supply, cosmetics, and products that emit radiation.

Folk medicine Traditional medicine practiced without a scientific understanding of the processes involved, usually handed down to the common people from earlier times.

General Adaptation Syndrome (GAS) The syndrome described by Hans Selye as the total organism's nonspecific response to stress.

Generativity versus Stagnation Erikson's psychosocial crisis from 40 to 65 years of age.

Health Insurance Portability and Accountability Act of 1996 (HIPAA) Government rules, regulations, and procedures resulting from legislation designed to protect the confidentiality of patient information.

Hierarchy Arranged to a specific order or rank; sequential arrangement.

High-context communication Communication style that involves great reliance on body language, reference to objects in the environment, and culturally relevant phraseology to convey an idea. Relies on the listener knowing related events through close association with the speaker or culture.

Homeostasis State of balance within the internal environment of the body.

Hospice An interdisciplinary program of palliative care and supportive services that addresses the physical, spiritual, social, and economic needs of terminally ill clients and their families. This care may be provided in the home or a hospice center.

Hypomania Mild form of mania with elevated elation and hyperactivity.

Id A person's basic animal nature; it is unconscious and amoral.

Identity versus Role Confusion Erikson's psychosocial crisis from 12 to 18 years of age.

Industry versus Inferiority Erikson's psychosocial crisis from 6 to 11 years of age.

Initiative versus Guilt Erikson's psychosocial crisis from 3 to 6 years of age.

Instrumental conditioning Learned response through reinforcement. Also known as *operant conditioning*.

***International Classification of Diseases-Clinical Modification* (ICD-CM)** Standard diagnosis codes used to identify a client's medical problem.

Intimacy versus Isolation Erikson's psychosocial crisis from 19 to 40 years of age.

Intimate partner violence (IPV) Physical, sexual, or psychological/emotional violence directed toward a spouse or former spouse, current or former partner, or current or former dating partner.

Kinesics Study of the body and its static and dynamic position as a means of communication.

Landau reflex When an infant is held in the prone position, the entire body forms a convex upward arc.

Life-altering illness An illness that affects or limits the quality of life. Some chronic illnesses and most life-threatening illnesses are life-altering illnesses.

Locomotion Ability to move from one place to another; hitch and pull self for movement.

Low-context communication Communication style that utilizes few environmental or cultural idioms to convey an idea or concept. Ideas are spelled out explicitly.

Mania Extreme periods of excitement, euphoria, delusions and hyperactivity followed by extreme lows of depression.

Moxibustion TCM technique that places a small amount of a spongy herb (mugwort) on a cone-shaped device and burned creating heat to promote healing.

Operant conditioning Learned response through reinforcement. Also known as *instrumental conditioning*.

Palliative Relieving or alleviating without curing.

Parasympathetic nervous system The craniosacral division of the autonomic nervous system.

Perceptions The images people have in their minds of places, situations, or events. Perceptions may differ from reality.

Pleasure principle Immediate gratification or primitive drives; whatever satisfies an impulse is good and whatever blocks or frustrates it is bad.

Polygenic Genetic trait determined by a group of genes.

Postconventional level The first level of Kohlberg's theory on moral development. Individuals' ethical principles are guided by consequences.

Preconventional level Kohlberg's theory that punishment and reward are understood. To do good is to avoid punishment.

Prejudice The process of "prejudging" something, usually in a biased manner.

Preoperational Period Piaget's cognition period from 2 to 6 years of age.

Projection Attributing one's own thoughts or impulses to another individual as if they had originated in the other person.

Psychoneuroimmunology The study of how the mind affects health and disease resistance.

Psychosis Mental disorder in which thoughts and emotions are so impaired that contact with reality is lost.

Psychosocial crises Conflicts between a person and society or social institutions.

Qigong Similar to tai chi, qigong is a series of postures, breathing techniques, and focused attention to promote healing and balance and increase vitality.

Rationalization The mind's way of justifying behavior by offering an explanation that is other than a truthful response.

Reality principle That which exists; what is real.

Regionalism Speech or manners representative of a specific geographical location.

Regression An attempt to go back to an earlier stage of development to escape fear, anxiety, or conflict.

Repression Mind's way of forgetting or experiencing temporary amnesia until it can cope with an overwhelming circumstance.

Self-awareness Knowing oneself as an individual.

Sensorimotor Period Piaget's cognition period from birth to 2 years of age.

Social media Forms of electronic communication such as Web sites or blogs that enable users to share content or to participate in social networking, sharing ideas, and personal messages.

Sodomy Anal intercourse.

Stalking Repeated behavior causing someone high levels of fear.

Stereotyping The habit of attaching an uncomplimentary or generalized label to a person, race, idea, or the like.

Stress State of mental or emotional strain resulting from physical, physiological, or psychological stressors.

Stressors Stimuli, environmental factors, or life events that result in physiological arousal or stress.

Sublimation Redirecting a socially unacceptable impulse into socially acceptable behavior.

Subluxation Partial vertebrae misalignment (chiropractic theory)

Substance Use Disorder (SUD) Substance abuse and addiction.

Superego The moral branch of the personality; the ideal self that strives for perfection.

Suppression Deliberately refusing to acknowledge something that causes mental pain or suffering.

Sympathetic nervous system The thoracolumbar division of the autonomic nervous system.

Trust versus Mistrust Erikson's psychosocial crisis from birth to 18 months of age.

Undoing To cancel out a behavior or to try to make amends.

Unresolved grief Grief that lasts longer than most individual's experience or for their cultural background.

Western medicine A term used to describe allopathic medicine, orthodox medicine, or the way medicine has traditionally been practiced in the United States and Europe. Western medicine utilizes the scientific method and employs pharmaceuticals combined with surgical procedures to combat disease and illness.

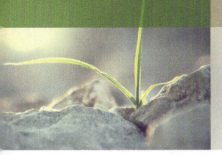

Index

(‘b’ indicates boxed material; ‘i’ indicates an illustration; ‘t’ indicates a table)